Praise for
The New Truth About Menopause

"Just when we need it most, Landau and Cyr have taken the guesswork out of navigating the maze of scientific information on menopause and available treatments. They have sorted through the most recent research on symptom management and disease-prevention options and compiled it into an exceptionally clear, useful, interesting, and fun resource for women confronted with treatment decisions."

—Nananda Col, M.D., Assistant Professor of Medicine,
Division of Women's Health, Harvard Medical School

"Landau and Cyr have shed new light on the myths of menopause. *The New Truth About Menopause* confirms that there is more to midlife than only menopause. Especially useful are the graphs, decision-making tools, and the profiles of real women that sound like 'us' but individualized for special needs."

—Diana Taylor, R.N., Ph.D., coauthor of
*Taking Back the Month: A Personalized Solution for Managing PMS
and Enhancing Your Health*

"This book is a great resource to help women maintain health and vitality during menopause. Readers are taught about the Stages of Change for enhancing life through behavior change. The latest evidence is provided to help women make informed decisions, including whether hormone therapy is right for them."

—Janice M. Prochaska, M.S.W., Ph.D.,
president and CEO of Pro-Change Behavior Systems, Inc.

. . . and for
The Complete Book of Menopause

"Without a doubt this is the best book on menopause available. My patients and I have been waiting for a book like this: scientifically sound, positive and balanced in perspective, written with intelligence and wit. The authors, leaders in the women's health field, have drawn on their rich clinical and personal experience to produce a positive, practical, intelligent guide to menopause."

—Karen J. Carlson, M.D.,
Harvard Medical School

"This compassionate and empowering resource deserves a place on every woman's shelf."

—Karen Johnson, M.D., Department of Psychiatry,
University of California, San Francisco, and
cofounder of the Women's Health Project

"The first comprehensive handbook to offer clear, detailed, and reassuring information on every aspect of this stage of life."

—*Women's Health Digest*

"A treasure chest of information on the health and well-being of women. Menopause is mysterious and intimidating for many women. This book removes the mystery and shows how women can be happy and healthy during this time of life."

—Kelly Brownell, Ph.D., Professor of Psychology, Yale University

"A truly comprehensive book for this stage of life. Conversational yet authoritative. Excellent lists of resources and references."

—*Harvard Women's Health Watch*

"The authors have written a book that beautifully captures the essence of women's health. It should be required reading for all physicians."

—John Noble, M.D., Chief of General Internal Medicine, Boston City Hospital

The New Truth About Menopause

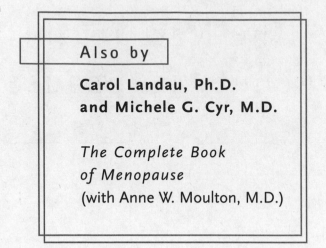

Also by

**Carol Landau, Ph.D.
and Michele G. Cyr, M.D.**

*The Complete Book
of Menopause*
(with Anne W. Moulton, M.D.)

The New Truth About Menopause

Straight Talk About Treatments and Choices from Two Leading Women Doctors

CAROL LANDAU, PH.D.

MICHELE G. CYR, M.D.

St. Martin's Griffin ✦ New York

www.stmartins.com

Design by Alamini Design

LIBRARY OF CONGRESS CATALOGING-IN-PUBLICATION DATA

Landau, Carol.
    The new truth about menopause : straight talk about
treatments and choices from two leading women doctors /
by Carol Landau and Michele G. Cyr.— 1st U.S. ed.
       p. cm.
    Includes resources (p. 153) and index (p. 183).
    ISBN 0-312-31798-0
    1. Menopause—Popular works. 2. Middle-aged women—
Health and hygiene—Popular works. I. Cyr, Michele G.
II. Title.
RG186.L363 2003
618.1'75—dc21

2003047152

10 9 8 7 6 5 4 3 2

*To David and Rob
and
Greg and Ben*

Authors' Note

The contents of this work are intended to further understanding and discussion only and are not intended and should not be relied upon as recommending or promoting a specific diagnosis or treatment for any particular person. In view of ongoing research, changes in governmental regulations, and the constant flow of information relating to the use of medication, the reader is urged to consult with her own health care professional and to review and evaluate the information provided in the package insert or instructions for each medication. The fact that a publication, organization, or Web site is referred to in this work as a citation and/or a potential source of further information does not mean that the authors endorse all of the information the organization or Web site may provide or recommendations it may make. Further, readers should be aware that Internet Web sites listed in this work may have changed or disappeared between when this work was written and when it is read. The names and identifying characteristics in all case studies have been changed.

Table of Contents

The New Truth About Menopause

CHAPTER ONE

The New Truth About Menopause

"Don't panic! You will be okay. Let's rethink this." This is the beginning of many conversations we've had with our understandably anxious patients after they saw the alarming front-page headlines in 2002 about the dangers of hormone therapy. The Women's Health Initiative (WHI), a federally funded study, released a statement that it was stopping its trial of estrogen plus progestin because enough data had been collected to conclude that the long-term risks of the hormones outweighed the benefits. The increased risk of breast cancer, which had long been feared, was now well documented. There were increases in blood clots and strokes as well. But the real surprise, after years of reports that hormone treatment helped protect women against heart disease, was that there were no heart benefits to offset these negative consequences. So the millions of women in the United States who were taking hormone therapy woke up to quotes in the *New York Times* like, "This [estrogen/progestin] is a dangerous drug," from Dr. Deborah Grady, a well-respected leader in women's health. The second-largest selling drug in the United States was suddenly suspect, and the women taking it were overwhelmed by fear and distrust.

While discussing this bombshell we asked, "Could this situation get any *more* frightening?" Well, in fact it could and it did. The next week, the *Journal of the American Medical Association* published more upsetting news: a possible link between estrogen therapy and ovarian cancer. Breast cancer, as terrifying as it is, can often be detected early by breast exams and mammograms, but ovarian cancer is a notorious silent killer of women. Even though this was a single study, all hell broke loose. Midlife women, once promised estrogen as a magic bullet, were stunned.

In May 2003, after much of the menopause news had quieted down, additional analyses from the Women's Health Initiative were released. As one professor of gynecology told the Associated Press, there was "another nail in the coffin for the use of hormones during and after menopause." The lead article in the *Journal of the American Medical Association* revealed even more unexpected results from the WHI. Many experts had believed, again based on earlier uncontrolled studies, that estrogen might prevent Alzheimer's disease and improve cognitive functioning in older women. A subset of women participating in the WHI were evaluated specifically to determine whether the combination of estrogen and a progestin would prevent Alzheimer's disease and other types of dementia. Dementia is a larger category that includes Alzheimer's disease and other causes of impairment in memory, judgment, and reasoning. Once again, the surprise was that women taking hormone therapy (after age sixty-five—the age of the women in the study) were *more*, not less, likely to develop Alzheimer's disease or other forms of dementia.

Further analysis of the breast cancers that were diagnosed in the WHI participants revealed some troubling results. The breast cancers that were diagnosed in women taking estrogen plus progestin were slightly larger and more likely to have spread to lymph nodes and beyond. Previous studies had suggested that although hormone therapy might increase the risk of breast cancer, the breast cancers that developed on hormones had a better prognosis. This new information from the WHI contradicts that prior thinking. The study implies that there was a delay in the detection in spite of yearly mammograms and breast exams. An additional finding was that the women on combined hormone therapy were much more likely to have abnormal mammograms after only one year of treatment, and this increase continued throughout the five years of study.

After the Women's Health Initiative results were released, and so many women were upset and confused, some physicians said that they just stopped answering their phones. "Nice," we thought. After having a clear preference for using estrogen for decades, they retreated into silence now that the situation had become complicated.

We decided to take the opposite approach, to communicate with as many people as quickly as possible. We know that midlife women today need both an update on information as well as a plan for making new decisions. *The New Truth About Menopause* is the result of our many conversations with patients, family members, friends, and colleagues. We wrote this book to calm your fears if you are worried about the decisions you've made in the past and confused about decisions you need to make in the future. Drawing on our many years of experience in women's health and menopause education, the book establishes a process for making informed choices about menopause. It will empower you by reducing your anxiety and clarifying your options.

The outlook is brighter than you might think. Consider the following:

- There was never only one good option for treating the symptoms of menopause. Each woman has a specific history and medical risks that should be considered before making any choices.
- Menopause may lead to many health decisions or few. It all depends on your individual symptoms, medical problems, lifestyle, and needs.
- You have many more choices than you may realize. For every condition that estrogen was supposed to treat, there are other effective, safe, and well-tolerated medications and strategies, and new medications and herbal preparations are being developed at a rapid pace.
- If you are currently taking hormone therapy, you can think through your decision. It may be that in your particular situation, the benefits are worth the risks. We will help you re-evaluate your choices and discuss them with your health care professional.
- Lifestyle changes can result in enormous benefits to your health.

- There are millions of midlife women, so you are never alone with these concerns.

This last point raises an important issue: It's time to dispense with the negativism that pervades so many discussions of the whole topic. Almost every book or popular article on menopause has an undercurrent of pessimism and dread. Yes, menopause is a sign that we are growing older, and in our youth-oriented culture, this is dangerous territory. But guess what? We can grow older and try to do so with good health, good relationships, and wisdom. Or we can die young. If these are our choices, let's choose Door No. 1.

Midlife, then, is a target for our worst fears. Much of the hype about menopause has been a thinly veiled sales promotion for estrogen and other menopausal cures. In addition to aging, menopause represents a fear of death, of loss of control and femininity. Many of the major popular books have fueled these fears and overemphasized the positive effects of estrogen. Gail Sheehy's *The Silent Passage*, for example, paid enormous attention to physical appearance and extolled the power of estrogen. "I was staggered by the potency of the feminine hormone."

Television programs are even worse. Archie Bunker, in the groundbreaking *All in the Family* series in the 1970s, demanded that his wife, Edith, go through menopause quickly. Edith had been even more upset and tearful than usual. "If you're gonna have a change of life, you gotta do it right now. I'm gonna give you just thirty seconds." Many of the complaints about women's menopause are similarly male-oriented. In the 1960s, Dr. Robert Wilson wrote an extraordinarily influential book, *Feminine Forever*, that promised, "Estrogen makes women adaptable, even-tempered and generally easy to live with." Unbeknownst to his readers, Dr. Wilson was backed by a foundation supported in part by Wyeth-Ayerst Pharmaceuticals, the makers of one of the earliest estrogen medications, Premarin. His foundation published the book, which was effectively a marketing tool for estrogen.

Menopause also feeds into our competition with other women. From an early age, as women we learn to compare and compete with other women. Who is thinner? Prettier? Bigger-breasted? More popular? And of course, who looks younger? We've heard men and women alike suggest that any woman over 35 is "menopausal." Two decades after *All in the Family,* the supposedly women-oriented television series *Sisters* included a younger woman played by actress Sela Ward, who got revenge on an older, competitive colleague by suggesting that she "has had such a difficult menopause."

Even one of the many post–Women's Health Initiative articles on menopause, written by a women's health physician, used the following words loaded with negative emotions: "vanishing eggs," "ovarian failure," "the aging ovary," "calcium pours out of bones," "the withering of reproductive organs," and the latest negative term for menopause, "reproductive senescence." Notice the intensity, the nonclinical nature of these descriptions. Men's problems don't get addressed with this same negativity. One never reads about, for example, the "withering penis" or "desperately plunging levels of testosterone" when men write about erectile or sexual dysfunction.

In the past, these negative terms were used to propel women toward using the magic bullet, hormone therapy. As it turns out, the bullet never was magic. It was a medication that, like all medications, had risks and benefits.

We believe that you can take charge of your health and your life and that not all changes or symptoms require treatment. A medical model—underwritten not only by a sincere belief in estrogen but also by hormone therapy marketing campaigns—has overdramatized the challenges of menopause. Midlife comes to us all, and there have always been older women who are healthy and happy. And now, as you'll see, there is an explosion of new treatments. Remember, too, that each of us is unique. No two women have exactly the same pattern of symptoms or long-term concerns at menopause. If you are like most women, you'll be able to deal with your lot. After all, it's not the end of the world; it's just the end of your periods.

So let's get started. We find it helpful to begin with a shared vocabulary. Here are some basic menopause definitions and facts:

- Menopause is the normal developmental stage that occurs after a woman's last menstrual period.
- Menopause is usually diagnosed when a woman hasn't had a period for twelve months or when a blood test indicates it.

- A blood test measuring FSH (follicle-stimulating hormone) can also diagnose menopause. A high level of FSH (above 40) indicates menopause. Since FSH stimulates the ovaries to make estrogen, the pituitary is on overdrive when estrogen levels decline, producing more FSH. In other words, when estrogen is low, FSH is high.
- The average age of menopause is 51 years (51.4 years, to be exact).
- For 95 percent of women, menopause occurs any time between 40 and the late 50s. When menopause occurs before age 40, it is called premature. This could be a result of a medical problem, so it definitely should be evaluated by your health care professional.
- Perimenopause is the time before menopause when menstruation becomes irregular. It lasts approximately four years, but each woman's experience is different.
- Hot flashes are by far the most common symptom of menopause.
- Night sweats are hot flashes that occur at night and involve profuse sweating. They can disrupt sleep.
- Another common change is the thinning and dryness of the vaginal wall. This sometimes leads to discomfort and irritation.
- Estrogen is an umbrella term for the female hormones used to treat the symptoms of menopause. It is available in different types and in many forms. At one time its use was referred to as ERT, or estrogen replacement therapy. Now the term estrogen therapy (ET) is used. The most common form of estrogen is conjugated equine estrogen, Premarin, first introduced in 1942 and so named because it is derived from pregnant mares' urine. Forty-five million prescriptions for Premarin were written in 2001.
- Progestin is the name used for a wide range of hormones that have the properties of progesterone, which is also produced during the menstrual cycle. A progestin is added to estrogen, unless a woman has had a hysterectomy. This is done because estrogen used alone leads to a buildup on the wall of the uterus, or endometrial hyperplasia, that can lead to uterine cancer. Estrogen plus a progestin was often called combined hormone replacement therapy, or HRT. Now the term hormone therapy (HT) or estrogen plus progestin (EPT) is used.

Let's use these terms and facts to answer some basic questions: What causes menopause? What are the main effects of menopause? What can I do about these effects? We'll also debunk some of the most common myths about menopause.

What Causes Menopause?

Menopause is the third natural major reproductive phase in a woman's life. Each baby girl is born with millions of immature eggs in her ovaries. The actual number of eggs is genetically determined. Recent studies, for example, have identified a gene that is associated with early menopause. That gene is associated with a woman having fewer eggs at birth. By the time a girl reaches menarche, the time when her menstrual cycles begin, the number of eggs is already reduced. The cause is unclear. Each month an egg is developed, but approximately 1,000 eggs will be shed. The follicles surrounding the eggs produce the ovaries' hormone, estrogen. If a sperm fertilizes an egg, pregnancy takes place. This causes another set of hormonal changes.

Usually, when a woman reaches her late 40s, her FSH level goes up and periods become shorter or unpredictable. The hallmark of the transition to menopause is the change in menstrual cycles. These changes involve the length of a period, the intensity of the flow, and the number of days in the menstrual cycle. Most women have four to eight years of menstrual changes before menopause actually occurs. Some women, on the other hand, just notice that their periods have stopped. These changes are the natural results of the declining levels of estrogen.

(A word of caution, however: Unusual or abnormal uterine bleeding is a different story. If your bleeding is much heavier than usual or lasts more than seven days or if you have blood clots or anemia, you should promptly consult your physician. In addition, bleeding or spotting after intercourse or between periods can also be cause for concern.)

So menstrual changes signify the beginning of perimenopause, the entrée into the transition. Then hello, hot flashes! When menopause occurs, around age 51, estrogen production from the ovaries, or estradiol, is reduced by 90 percent. However, estrone, which is produced and stored in fat cells, replaces estradiol. Environmental and behavioral conditions can also hasten menopause. Smoking can bring on menopause years earlier than it would occur normally. Some chemical exposures can lead to an earlier menopause. Radiation therapy and chemotherapy can also cause menopause. And of course, when the ovaries are surgically removed, menopause occurs immediately.

Now we can go on, as psychoanalytic theorists did, to bemoan this loss of reproductive phase of a woman's life. Helene Deutsch, for example, wrote that a woman lost "her service to the species." Many psychoanalytic thinkers used this belief to explain what they saw as a natural, almost preordained midlife depression, termed involutional melancholia. Unfortunately, their belief system led to an overestimate of depression in midlife women and inattention to the much more prevalent depressions in younger women.

But there is another view, based more in reality. Many women struggle with birth control during their reproductive years. Some women experience mood swings associated with their menstrual cycles, the PMS for which we women are also often blamed or ridiculed. Other women are troubled by infertility in their 30s and 40s. The main infertility support group is called Resolve, suggesting that couples should do what they can and then come to peace with their situation, whatever it may be. And of course, many women give birth or adopt children. So perhaps by the time we reach our 50s we have not come to ovarian failure but to another type of resolution. Maybe, as Mary Mahowald, an ethicist, has suggested, we have reached ovarian fulfillment or ovarian completion syndrome. And remember, we women are not primarily reproductive organs, but rather complex individuals who happen to have female reproductive systems.

In fact, many women do associate menopause with reproductive freedom. And there is a long history of differing perceptions of menopause. For example, in 1818, the U.S. attorney general, William Wirt, had an inquiry for the family physician. It seemed that Mr. Wirt's wife, Elizabeth, was not becoming pregnant.

In Anya Jobour's *Marriage in the Early Republic* we get a glimpse of Elizabeth's views on the subject. Earlier in their marriage, Elizabeth Wirt responded to a teasing question from her husband as to whether she was pregnant, to which she responded, "With me—as there is no prospect of escape—I only wish that when it must come I might have some choice in the affair." By the end of her letter, however, Elizabeth Wirt backs down by adding, "These things are overruled by Providence, and our part is cheerful submission" (p. 75). Later, although Mr. Wirt was unhappy, his wife was not. Elizabeth Wirt wrote to her mother that she was overjoyed at the situation because by 1818 she had already given birth to her twelfth child.

What Are Menopausal Symptoms?

The primary symptoms of menopause are hot flashes and changes in the urinary and sexual organs and functioning. There are also less direct and less severe changes in mood and thinking (cognition), but these have been exaggerated as direct effects of estrogen loss. All the other symptoms—skin changes, memory loss, gray hair, and wrinkles—are part of the aging process and less directly related to menopause. In other words, midlife men get them, too, and there is much less fuss about it.

Hot Flashes

These are the calling card of menopause, or perimenopause to be exact. Somewhere between 75 and 85 percent of menopausal women in North America have them. Approximately 25 percent have hot flashes disturbing enough to seek treatment, and 15 percent find them to be severe. A part of the brain called the hypothalamus regulates body temperature. Some experts believe that changes in this temperature control mechanism cause hot flashes.

A hot flash seems to come out of nowhere. It begins with an overwhelming sensation of heat, followed by sweating, and is sometimes accompanied by heart palpitations. Then just as suddenly, body temperature drops, leaving a woman shivering and cold. Night sweats can significantly disrupt sleep, with these wide swings in temperature lending to multiple changes of nightclothes and bed linens. The severity of hot flashes varies from woman to woman. Similarly, some women may have them for several months, whereas others may have them for many years.

Here is how a hot flash happens. The capillaries in the skin suddenly open wider. This leads to blood rushing in, a flush, and pores opening. When the capillaries contract, the blood drains away, body temperature drops, and the skin pales. For some women, a hot flash is a not unpleasant sensation of warmth. For others, especially women after an oophorectomy (the surgical removal of one's ovaries) or chemotherapy, hot flashes can be disruptive and severe. In addition, some women experience a sense of dread just before a hot flash, with anxiety during and after. We'll explore treatments for hot flashes in detail in Chapter 3. Briefly, however, the main choices are estrogen, progestin, antidepressants, blood pressure medications, herbal remedies, soy, and self-management strategies. So you see, you have a lot of treatments to consider.

Sexual and Urinary Symptoms

Hot flashes and irregular periods are the first symptoms of perimenopause. Later, about five years after menopause, vaginal dryness may become noticeable. This can lead to an uncomfortable burning feeling, and sexual intercourse can be painful. Once again, however, we can thank the estrogen promoter Dr. Robert Wilson and others who referred to menopause as "a horror of living decay" for exaggerating this condition. Just to help out, Dr. David Reuben, of *Everything You Always Wanted to Know About Sex* fame, described menopause as a time of "decline of breasts and female genitalia." And it is true that the female sexual organs depend in part on estrogen to maintain their anatomy and function. But please! In reality, the decrease in estrogen levels at the time of menopause does not lead to irreparable, inevitable, or disastrous changes.

There are treatments for vaginal symptoms, too. In addition to low-dose vaginal estrogen, there are moisturizers. Sheryl Kingsberg, a psychologist at Case Western Reserve Medical School, was quoted in a news article about menopause: "We shy away from even discussing vaginal moisturizers. We feel comfortable using moisturizer for our face to prevent dry skin. This is the same thing." In addition, she and most experts agree that when it comes to sex, more is more. Practice makes perfect, or in this case, practice makes pleasure. "I like to think of it as going to the gym. Once I'm on the treadmill I think, This is great. I'm coming back again soon." Comparing sex to a workout on the treadmill may not be very arousing, but you get the basic idea.

Many women complain of memory loss and mood swings. In general, mood swings are associated with perimenopause, especially in women who have hot flashes. As is true for women of all ages, high levels of stress and other medical problems can lead to depression. Women who have histories of depression may be vulnerable for a recurrence at the time of menopause. But most women should expect transient moodiness, not unlike milder cases of PMS.

As for memory changes, estrogen may well affect verbal memory. This could be true because estrogen may influence the brain chemicals known as neurotransmitters that assist in learning. Once again, for women going through natural menopause, memory changes are not severe. However, more significant changes are seen in women who have had their ovaries surgically removed (oophorectomies) or experienced sudden menopause due to chemotherapy or radiation therapy.

The Importance of Prevention

Those are, simply, the major symptoms associated with menopause. Midlife is also a time when women begin to focus on preventing conditions associated with menopause and aging. Some of the major conditions to consider are osteoporosis, heart disease, Alzheimer's disease, and most cancers. While most cancers are not specifically related to menopause, many do become more common with age. A few, such as breast cancer, are associated with some treatments that we'll discuss later.

Osteoporosis

The loss of estrogen at menopause interferes with the normal process of building and maintaining bones. Over time, bones can thin, leading to osteoporosis. Up to 20 percent of bone mass can be lost during the first five to ten years after menopause. Osteoporosis is a serious condition.

After menopause, almost half of all women will suffer some type of fracture due to osteoporosis. Even more troubling is that 20 percent of women die within one year of suffering a hip fracture. Clearly, we want to prevent this condition.

The two basics of an osteoporosis prevention plan are adequate intake of calcium—1,200 to 1,500 milligrams a day, with 400 IU (International Units) of vitamin D—and maintaining good bone strength with weight-bearing exercise. Other treatments that we'll present in Chapter 4 include bisphosphonates (Fosamax, Actonel, or Didronel), raloxifene (Evista), or calcitonin (Miacalcin), estrogen, and many new medications in the pipeline.

Heart Disease

Heart disease is the number one killer of women. We can do a lot to prevent it. At one time, the medical community was optimistic that estrogen prevented heart disease. With the results of the Women's Heath Initiative, however, it appears that the opposite may be true. This still leaves us with the options of a heart-healthy diet, exercise, medications to lower cholesterol and blood pressure, low-dose aspirin (81 milligrams per day), and moderate (only) intake of alcohol. We will give you details later.

Alzheimer's Disease

Alzheimer's disease is a condition that affects memory and brain functioning. It is a progressive and tragic disease. Alzheimer's is *not* the normal memory slippage that occurs with aging. Although research is ongoing, currently there is no definitive effective treatment.

Preliminary research had suggested that estrogen, especially when started early and taken for more than 10 years, might reduce the risk of developing Alzheimer's by as much as 50 percent. However, the randomized controlled study from the Women's Health Initiative found that women who were over the age of 65 and taking the combination hormone therapy were twice as likely to develop Alzheimer's disease and other types of dementia than those taking a placebo. Given the current risks of hormone therapy, estrogen plus progestin should not be prescribed to prevent dementia. This is definitely an area of active research to watch.

Menopause Myths

Now that you are armed with these basics, we also need to dispel some all-too-common myths:

Myth 1 *Menopause is a disease and must be treated medically.* Not true. On the other hand, there is no need to suffer unnecessarily because of a belief that menopause is totally natural. Although the decrease in estrogen can lead to troubling symptoms and to osteoporosis, it is a natural, gradual transition. Most women adjust to the declining estrogen levels within a few years.

Myth 2 *Any remedy labeled "natural" is better or harmless.* First of all, there is no regulation of the term natural. In addition, herbal products are not held to the same standards as medications approved for use by the Food and Drug Administration (FDA). In order for a medication to be approved by the FDA to treat a specific condition, studies must be conducted to demonstrate its effectiveness. The research also documents side effects and contraindications, which are made available to health care professionals and the public. In contrast, an herbal product is regulated only in a general way. So not only can companies make false claims for herbal products, they are not required to test side effects or interactions with medications. We say, be careful.

Myth 3 *Most women become depressed at the time of menopause.* This is a tricky one but is also false. Some women do become moody, but more often during perimenopause, not after menopause. Sleep deprivation may be the culprit some of the time. Most experts agree that untreated night sweats can lead to sleep deprivation, and this lack of sleep can trigger a depressive episode in a small group of women.

More often, such stressful life events as poor overall health, the death of a spouse or partner, or the need to care for elderly family members are associated with depression and anxiety. Studies of midlife women found that these stresses, not changes in hormones, predicted depression in most women, though the story may be different for women who have histories of depression, especially postpartum depression or late luteal phase depression (depression associated with PMS).

Other women are unsettled by mood swings. Again, mood swings occur more often during perimenopause and are time-limited. Since antidepressant medication can treat both depressed mood and hot flashes, there is even more hope here.

Myth 4 *Menopause can make you crazy.* Well, on the one hand, if we took any individual, deprived her of sleep, and subjected her to dozens of hot flashes and night sweats every day for many months, we could understand that she could become irrational, irritable, and unproductive! However, if we take severe hot flashes out of the equation, menopause is merely a stage in life, and like other phases, has its ups and downs.

Why do we all hear so many stories about someone's Aunt Matilda who was up in the attic ranting and raving? Well, some psychiatric conditions, if untreated, get worse over time. Sometimes loss, illness, and the stresses of midlife and aging can cause severe psychological reactions in both men and women. But in addition, our society is particularly harsh on midlife and older women. Images and stereotypes of evil and crazy older women are pervasive, from the old witches in fairy tales to the Wicked Witch of the West in *The Wizard of Oz* and Cruella DeVil in the Disney film *101 Dalmatians*.

As women involved in menopause education, we pay close attention to media portrayals of crazy or depressed menopausal woman. In short, we collect menopause stories. Ten years ago our favorite was the menopause legal defense in the offbeat television program *Picket Fences*. Yet another menopausal woman had killed a man in some blinding hormonal frenzy. Recently an even more dramatic example occurred in the HBO series *The Sopranos*, when Carmela Soprano finally asked her husband, mob boss Tony Soprano, to leave. In discussing Carmela's decision with their daughter, Meadow, Tony says that Carmela is having a "hard time because of the change." Tony and Meadow both know that Carmela has suffered through Tony's numerous affairs, as well as his brutal and criminal behavior, yet she's trapped by their lavish lifestyle. Her crush on a low-level mobster ended when he left her without saying good-bye; and Meadow, a college student, has recently humiliated

Carmela at dinner during a discussion of a novel. Knowing all this, father and daughter back away from the reality. Meadow agrees, "Yes, it must be menopause." (But this scene does represent a breakthrough as well, since both characters seem to have some sense that they're using menopause as an excuse to avoid acknowledging the real sources of stress in Carmela's life.)

Myth 5 *Menopause signifies the end of a healthy sexual life.* This myth is also related to a misconception that women become masculinized by menopause. In reality, it is true that with aging, sexual arousal takes longer for both men and women. One view of this is that women are slower to arouse with age. Another view, however, is that women do not get enough stimulation to become aroused. The net result is that it takes longer for women to become lubricated during foreplay. The explanation for these changes are numerous, including decreased blood flow to the vagina, which makes it less sensitive to stimulation, and decreased vaginal lubrication related to estrogen levels. In some women, there may be a change in the experience of orgasm and a decrease in the frequency of orgasms after menopause. But you do not have to be one of them! Although sexual changes do occur as we grow older, with good communication, these need not interfere with a fulfilling sex life.

Myth 6 *Menopause is the beginning of the end.* Much of the marketing of treatments for menopause plays on our fear of aging. As mentioned earlier, Dr. Robert Wilson started this trend with his book promoting Premarin (despite a conflict of interest). In *Feminine Forever,* he warned women that only with estrogen, "Breasts and genitals will not shrivel." Other advertisers have followed suit. We've seen many other claims of "curing" everything from wrinkles to gray hair!

In reality, most women adjust quite well to the changes associated with menopause. For most women, midlife brings a sense of freedom, and for other women, the struggles are really about life and getting older, not some "menopausal syndrome."

There are decisions to be made, and to make the best decisions, we need to be free of fear. You can do this. You've undoubtedly made many health decisions before. Maybe you had acne as a young woman and chose a treatment. You've probably made choices about birth control, and too many of us have made many decisions about dieting. Most women have also either made health decisions for family members or helped them to do so. This is not all that different. We'll take it step by step to give you the skills to make health decisions now and in the future.

A Straightforward Model for Making Health Decisions

All too often, a woman goes to her physician's office and comes out with a prescription in hand. Yet she may not know why she should take the specific medication. She may not know the common side effects or even the more serious risks of the medication. She may not even *want* to take a medication.

We want to change this. Our goal is to help you establish a logical process for making health decisions. If you become more involved in making these decisions, you will feel more in control of your health and of your life in general. You will also be more committed to whatever plans you make, whether they involve taking a medication, losing weight, or exercising more. Your commitment and motivation will lead you to be more successful, and thus a positive cycle will be created. Here's how we will proceed.

First, let's take inventory. What are you most concerned about now and for the future? Are you having troublesome hot flashes? Mood swings? Are you concerned about your risks for heart disease? Osteoporosis? You'll need to consider your current health profile, the current pressing issues, and your concerns about your health in the future.

The next step is to set specific goals. What do you want to happen? Most women want relief from the troublesome symptoms of menopause. So you might have a goal of stopping night sweats or treating vaginal dryness. Another possibility is that you want to prevent certain conditions like osteoporosis or colon cancer. Maybe you want to build up your muscle strength.

Next you'll want to gather information about your options. In the next chapter we will help you understand women's health research; then in Chapter 3, we'll present the latest knowledge about the treatment of symptoms and diseases associated with menopause. We'll also let you know the best resources—Web sites, books, and pamphlets available to help you stay fully informed.

Check with your doctor or health care professional, too, to see what she or he recommends. Schedule an appointment to do this. (The right time for important conversations is not when you are on your back having a Pap smear or when the doctor is going out the door at the end of the appointment or when you or your doctor is overly stressed.)

We will detail the best communication strategies in Chapter 6, but here are some initial tips. Listen to your doctor's responses to your concerns. Ask questions if you don't understand something. Be sure the treatments target your own specific goals, not general goals that are supposed to apply to all women. If your doctor interrupts you, calmly restate your point. If you feel as though you're not being taken seriously, express your opinion directly. State your goals. You might want to jot down a list of questions and concerns to take with you. If you tend to get nervous, your emotions will interfere with your ability to communicate and to process information. So you might ask someone close to you—your husband, your partner, or a friend, for example—to accompany you.

Once you've formulated your plan, it's time to act. This plan may involve taking a medication or herbal preparation, consuming more calcium and less fat in your diet, and/or increasing your exercise. Give yourself some time to implement all the steps in your plan. Continue to monitor your symptoms or goals.

Next, take a step back and evaluate your plan. Are your hot flashes occurring less often or less intensely? Are you having side effects from a medication or herbal preparation? Call your doctor. She or he can tell you whether the side effects will lessen with time or whether you need to adjust your dose. Have you been able to exercise? If not, tinker with your plan in order to improve it.

Take Heart

Our work in women's health has given us an opportunity to meet thousands of midlife women. One of the ways we've formalized the give-and-take is through our menopause town meetings, which we have been holding for over ten years in a variety of settings. Initially, we would deliver formal presentations, but we soon learned that the audiences—who impressed us time and again with their sophistication as health consumers—wanted something different. So now we make very brief introductory comments and open the floor to the audience. We not only answer questions but find that the women learn from each other and derive support from their shared experiences.

We continue to be inspired by the energy, resilience, and courage of these women. Their experiences have deepened our commitment to providing women with in-depth knowledge. For it is the combination of knowledge, self-confidence, and a good relationship with a primary health care professional that leads to informed health decisions.

Making smart health decisions can give us all an increased sense of competence and control. There are so many aspects of life that are out of our hands—disease, loss, and tragedy. But at the same time, we also need to recognize what we *can* control. The same is true with respect to our health. We cannot control our genetic makeup or family history, but we can control our exercise, stress management, nutrition, and problematic habits, and we can control the process of making health decisions. We will help you do this, with information on women's health research and treatment and preventive strategies, and with stories about how women make decisions. And we'll alert you to future trends and developments in sections called "Keep Your Eye On." By the time you reach the end of this book, you'll be better able to make decisions and enjoy this time of your life.

CHAPTER TWO

○─●─○

The Rise and Fall of Estrogen:

Understanding Women's Health Research

At least once a week, you will hear about or read a summary of a new medical paper. Perhaps it's on the radio, in the television news, or on the science page of your local newspaper. The results may be exaggerated to create a good headline or sound bite. Unless you're listening to public radio or television, the details may be scarce. Sometimes the conclusions will be frightening. Given the resources of the Internet and your local library, you can find out more about any article. But understanding research isn't always easy. By reviewing the history of estrogen treatments and research over the past hundred years, we hope to give you some tools to understand the terminology and the different types of research methods.

Early Menopause Remedies

Menopause got its bad reputation during the nineteenth century. C.P.L. de Gardanne, a French physician, devoted over a hundred pages to a variety of symptoms and conditions that were supposedly a result of menopause. In *De la ménépausie ou l'age critique des femmes* (Menopause, The Critical Age of Women), published in 1816, de Gardanne set the stage for later writers and proponents of remedies for this horrible women's disease.

The publications of nineteenth-century America often viewed menopause in negative terms, especially if there was a potion or elixir to sell. The pamphlets of the time contained numerous testimonials from individuals who proclaimed the power of the product. Dr. R.V. Pierce was a quite successful doctor-entrepreneur from Buffalo, New York. He offered consultations that tended to result in the prescription of one of his many products—elixirs, pellets, and "vaginal tablets." His advertisements were not just for women, but he claimed special expertise in this area: "There is every reason that women should not trust their delicate constitutions in the hands of a non-skilled person." Dr. Pierce included numerous testimonials for his remedies, published in *The People's Common Sense Medical Adviser in Plain English* (World's Dispensary Printing Office and Bindery, Buffalo, 1895). Here is a typical letter:

> *Gentlemen—*
> *I suffered terribly . . . my monthlies would nearly always send me to bed; I would lose from two to four quarts of blood. I had womb trouble pretty bad and my bladder would trouble me nearly all the time, by continually wanting to urinate, with smart, burning pains. My husband gave me a bottle of Dr. Pierce's "Favorite Prescription." I took 19 bottles and now feel very well indeed.*
>
> > Your friend,
> > Mrs. Lulu Clark

It may seem easy to dismiss this as quaint or ridiculous, but if you use the Internet, watch television, or read magazines, you have been bombarded by testimonials, too. For example, consider all the before and after pictures of people who supposedly benefited from weight-loss products. Even though most of the scientific professions prohibit testimonials in the advertising of medical treatments, such testimonials have, sadly, become extremely popular. A federal agency issued a "buyer beware" memo to the public in 2002, specifically mentioning weight-loss claims that do not have to be substantiated in any way. Any author or health care professional can take anecdotal evidence or testimonial claims, write a book, or give a seminar about his or her treatment plan or product, and proclaim it as the most effective. These claims are not subject to the same standards as material published in scientific journals. Ironically, some of the most outrageous claims are the most financially successful.

Case reports, or anecdotal evidence, are observations of small numbers of patients with a particular condition. Many peer-reviewed journals—that is, publications in which articles are evaluated by experts in the field before being accepted for publication—include case reports to generate new ideas. Still, case reports can also be subject to bias, or preconceived notions that influence the findings. This is where the pervasive negative outlook on menopause comes into play. For example, in 1869, Dr. George H. Napheys published *The Physical Life of Woman*. Here is what Dr. Napheys saw in his midlife patients: "she is utterly wretched, without any obvious cause of wretchedness. . . . From the commencement of the change of life commences also the steady diminution of the sexual passions, and soon after they disappear. Sometimes, however, the reverse takes place. . . . This should be regarded with alarm. It is contrary to the design of nature." Fortunately, Dr. Napheys's remedies were relatively benign, including heat treatments, the wearing of flannel (benign only if hot flashes were not an issue!), and the avoidance of alcohol. Other potions at the time contained whopping amounts of alcohol and sometimes even cocaine. Dr. Napheys did give a woman hope for the future. "Once safely through the critical period, the woman has a better chance for long life and a green old age than the man of equal years. . . . With the sweet consciousness of duty performed, she is now prepared to assist others by intelligent advice, cheerful counsel, and tender offices." Exactly which conditions was he treating here? Remarkably, we will read similar words a century later.

By the way, men are not the only ones who reflect bias. Dr. Mary Melendy suggested, in 1903, that menopausal women should "elevate their spirit and the body will grow strong," but cautioned that "there should be as little indulgence in the sexual relation as possible, none at all being preferable" and added that this "is essential to the welfare of men, as of women."

The turn of the twentieth century led to an interest in ovarian extracts for hot flashes, with case reports appearing in 1897. In 1929, Edward Doisy in the United States and Adolf Butenandt in Germany isolated the hormone estrone in human urine from pregnant women. Doisy later won the Nobel Prize. In 1933, a researcher at McGill University in Canada, James B. Collip, received a patent for Emmenin (no, not the rapper) from the urine of pregnant women. In 1939, Ayerst, a predecessor of Wyeth, discovered that pregnant mares' urine contained water-soluble estrogen conjugate, and Premarin was introduced in the United States three years later.

The Food and Drug Administration was established in 1906, but not until 1937 was the law amended to require manufacturers to prove and test medications for safety. In 1942 the FDA approved Premarin, or conjugated equine estrogen, for the treatment of hot flashes and genital atrophy based on many clinical trials. This process compared the effectiveness of the medication to that of a placebo, an inert sugar pill. The FDA also monitors side effects and adverse effects.

In general, you should be skeptical about treatments that are not FDA-approved. If there are claims about effectiveness, you need to ask the question "Was there a placebo or control group?" This is especially important because hot flashes usually decrease by 20 to 30 percent just from a placebo.

The 1950s and 1960s saw a rise in the use of Premarin. In 1959, the vague and numerous symptoms of the nineteenth century formally became a "menopausal syndrome." Dr. Robert Greenblatt wrote that "the menopausal woman must be considered to be physiologic castrate and replacement therapy should be administered to everyone with evidence of an estrogen lack" (cited in Walsh, 1966). So much for individual symptom differences and patient empowerment! Apparently some concerns had been raised prior to 1959 regarding an increased risk of breast and cervical cancer. Dr. Greenblatt's paper downplayed the risk of cancer. He wrote: "Statistics provided by the U.S. Public Health Service and the Commonwealth of Massachusetts reveal that the death rate from carcinoma of the breast has not materially increased in the past thirty years" (Walsh, 1966), despite the introduction of estrogen into medical practice.

Nor were male physicians alone in the enthusiasm for estrogen. Such testimonials as Ann Walsh's *E.R.T.: The Pills to Keep Women Young* extolled the cosmetic and psychological as well as the medical powers of estrogen. These case reports fueled an excitement about estrogen that was reflected in women's magazines of the day. The legitimate effectiveness of estrogen in treating hot flashes, night sweats, and vaginal symptoms, as well as the enthusiasm of many physicians, led many physicians to an increased use of estrogen. Enter Dr. Robert Wilson. A gynecologist, Dr. Wilson wrote that he personally treated "thousands of women" with estrogen. With an enormous amount of imaginative passion, Wilson proclaimed that every woman given estrogen would be *Feminine Forever*, the title of his bestselling book published in 1966. Dr. Wilson had also written articles in academic journals, and he denied any cancer risks, without providing any data. In his book, Dr. Wilson went even further and asserted that estrogen *prevented* cancer (p. 207).

In addition, Dr. Wilson went well beyond any legitimate medical indications and became a crusader. Here are just a few of his best lines:

> Instead of being condemned to witness the death of their own womanhood during what should be their best years, they will remain fully feminine—physically and emotionally—for as long as they live [p. 15].

> It is barbaric to expect that today's woman—just because she lives longer—must tolerate castration [p. 58].

> The problem here is not merely one of "bitchiness," a trait by no means confined to a woman of a certain age or condition. The menopausal syndrome is based on an erratic disorientation of the woman's entire frame of mind, a combination of mixed ideas and unpredictable caprice [p. 102].

Dr. Wilson's condescending views of lower-income women were particularly harsh:

> She rarely has the inclination—let alone the time—to occupy herself with new interests. . . . So she gradually descends into a state of almost bovine passivity [pp. 102–103].

His demeaning of social support was equally hostile:

Such women gradually flock together in small groups of three or four. Not that they have anything to share, but their boredom and trivial gossip [p. 103].

You probably won't be surprised to learn that men fared better in *Feminine Forever*:

Men retain their sexuality until quite late in life [p. 152].

Man is, by nature, polygamous [p. 200].

The gracefully aging male—erect, sprightly, and capable . . . [p. 153]

Even premature ejaculation (a result of a "bored husband," p. 149) and aloof behavior were the woman's fault: "Clearly there is something wrong with him, but it is not likely to be a lack of hormones in a man . . . the man is simply bored. The fault may be a dull mind, a dull job, or a dull wife" (p.153).

But perhaps the ultimate example of viewing women's menopause through a man's eyes is Dr. Wilson's boasting about saving a woman's life. A man came to see him, you see, because his wife was "old and crabby . . . hits the bottle and . . . won't fix meals." Fortunately, the gallant Dr. Wilson treated the woman intensively with estrogen injections three times a week—because otherwise the man, who had contracted tuberculosis and was a member of an organized crime family, had planned to shoot his wife. The husband "quietly laid a .32 automatic on the edge of my desk," Dr. Wilson reported (pp. 92–94). Apparently calling the police was not in Dr. Wilson's repertoire.

As it turned out, Dr. Wilson had both bias and a conflict of interest that blinded him to any downside of hormones. The fact that several pharmaceutical companies funded the Wilson Research Foundation was not revealed at the time. So Dr. Wilson was by no means an objective observer.

The later chapters of his book reveal even more bias. For it is only there that Dr. Wilson reveals that his own mother had a difficult time during menopause. As a boy, he observed a woman's body being recovered from a reservoir. "Why had she drowned herself? 'Gone mad,' the

town gossips insisted. 'The change of life,' they added by way of explanation. That phrase again! And in bewildered innocence I made a
dreadful mental connection between the ripped body of the drowned
woman and my own mother. . . . But it may well be that the episode at
Ramsbottom Reservoir remained alive in my unconscious life, guiding
me toward the choice of my medical specialty" (p.197). Fortunately,
Dr. Wilson bounced back from this painful memory to remind the
reader how much he enjoyed his Mercedes 540K Cabriolet (p. 199).
He ended his book with a flourish: "We stand at a threshold . . . seen in
historic perspective, the technique of menopause prevention reaches
far beyond the scope of any single life."

What a strange book! Even by the standards of 1966, Dr. Wilson's
pronouncements are misogynist and pompous. If his own words had
been attributed to a midlife woman, he'd no doubt have pronounced her
"mad . . . due to the change." Nonetheless, medicine had now spilled
into the popular culture with the promise of feminine, happy, manage-
able women. Similarly, in Dr. David Reuben's bestseller, *Everything You
Always Wanted to Know About Sex, but Were Afraid to Ask,* the author was proclaimed on the back cover as "replacing ignorance with knowledge." Yet
here is what readers learned from him about menopause and estrogen in
the first edition of his book, published in 1969:

"What causes the change of life anyway? A defect in the evolution
of human beings" (p. 360). Later, he describes life without estrogen,
"As the estrogen is shut off a woman comes as close as she can to
being a man. . . . Increased facial hair, deepened voice, obesity . . . not
really a man but no longer a functional woman, these individuals live
in the world of intersex" (p. 365). So, according to Dr. Reuben, the
estrogen-deprived women were not invited to join the sexual revolu-
tion. In the 1970s, then, Premarin sales skyrocketed, popular magazines promoted estrogen's cosmetic powers, and by the mid-seventies,
almost half of menopausal women had used HRT for about five years.

But let's get back to science. In the 1970s, women's health research
was beginning to rely more on data than on rhetoric. In 1975, the *New
England Journal of Medicine* published two papers linking postmenopausal
estrogen use to an increased risk in uterine cancer. Increased risk does
not necessarily indicate causality, but simply an association or a correlation. An example: Let's say you go to a meeting of Alcoholics Anony-

mous (AA) and see a lot of people drinking coffee or smoking cigarettes. So going to an AA meeting is associated, or correlated, with drinking coffee and/or smoking. Does going to the AA meeting itself *cause* the coffee drinking and/or smoking? No. More likely, the act of quitting drinking, withdrawal, stress, the sight of others drinking coffee and smoking, and the availability of coffee and/or cigarettes all play a role.

Sometimes a correlation can simply be a mistake. For example, at one time it was reported that being lesbian was correlated with drinking alcohol to excess. So people began to speculate that something about being lesbian led to increased drinking. Later it came out that the authors found their subjects where? In lesbian bars. So that proved to be a false correlation.

Now, back to the association of estrogen with uterine cancer. In the example of the studies reported in the 1975 *New England Journal of Medicine*, since the risk of uterine (endometrial) cancer was fourteen times greater for women who took estrogen alone, further investigation was warranted. It became clear that estrogen taken alone led to a buildup of the uterine lining called endometrial hyperplasia, a precursor to uterine cancer. Doctors at New York University found that adding medroxyprogesterone actetate (no wonder they call it MPA, trade name Provera), a progestin, eliminated the additional risk of endometrial cancer.

Around the same time, in 1976, a paper was published that suggested an increased risk of breast cancer in women taking estrogen. The association of estrogen use with cancer caused sales to drop. In the 1980s, however, the FDA approved another use for estrogen—to prevent the development of osteoporosis. By then, combination HT (estrogen plus progestin) was recommended to eliminate the risk of uterine cancer. Since the link with breast cancer was unclear, HT was viewed once again as a preventative long-term medication, especially since, at that time, there weren't many effective alternatives for the prevention of osteoporosis. Sales took off again.

The Role of Observational Studies

These are studies in which large groups of people are observed and specific symptoms and outcomes are measured. These studies have the advantage of using consistent measures and often involve huge numbers of subjects. Some of them are longitudinal studies, those that take place over a long period of time and can thus observe and track the development of certain symptoms and conditions. In observational studies, however, subjects are not randomly assigned to any treatment plan, but are simply observed in their everyday environment. We like to think of them as free-range people. With respect to menopause, observational studies led researchers to wonder whether estrogen had a protective effect on the heart. Several of these studies compared the women who took estrogen to those who did not. The studies showed that women taking estrogen tended to develop less heart disease than those who didn't.

By the 1970s, estrogen, in the form of Premarin, had been around for over thirty years, and its benefits and risks were becoming better understood. At first, observational studies were analyzed. The investigators had compared the heart disease risk of women who took estrogen with that of those who did not. To overcome some of the problems with this type of study, the researchers accounted for such important factors as cigarette smoking, high blood pressure, diabetes, elevated cholesterol levels, and obesity before doing comparisons. The investigators tried to make the groups as similar as possible, in terms of everything except their estrogen use.

The most famous of these observational studies is the Nurses' Health Study, established first by Dr. Frank Spitzer in 1976 and, in its second form, by Dr. Walter Willett of the Harvard Medical School and the Harvard School of Public Health in 1989. The goal of this enormous study, which represented the collaborative efforts of 80 physicians, other health care professionals, and epidemiologists, was to try to identify the risk factors for major chronic diseases of women, including cardiovascular disease. For example, one article reported on a survey of almost 122,000 female nurses between the ages of 30 and 55. The women completed questionnaires every two years. The questionnaires dealt with risk factors for cancer and heart disease. One report was published in the *New England Journal of Medicine* in 1985, and included information on hormone use and other possible risk factors. The conclusion of this study and several others was that postmenopausal use of estrogen reduced the risk of coronary artery disease. These results were impressive because of the large number of subjects involved.

But what could be wrong with drawing conclusions from the Nurses' Health and other observational studies? There were several potential problems. First, what if the women were different in ways other than those the investigators chose to examine? In that case, was the lower rate of cardiovascular disease a result of those differences rather than of the hormone therapy? Couldn't it be true, for example, that those women who were generally healthier were prescribed hormone therapy by their physicians? Was it possible that the women who chose to take hormone therapy exercised more than those who did not? Were doctors more likely to diagnose a woman with heart disease if she wasn't on estrogen? Dr. Elizabeth Barrett-Connor recently suggested that since the *Physicians' Desk Reference* of the period recommended that hormone therapy not be prescribed to women with heart disease, this might explain some of the findings of the Nurses' Health Study.

Nonetheless, the large numbers of women in this study and a high level of statistical significance led people to begin to link estrogen use with a reduced risk of heart disease. Statistical significance answers the question "Could the outcome have occurred by chance alone?" Statistical significance means that the findings of the study are unlikely to have occurred by chance. The conventional cutoff point is called a probability, or p-value, of less than .05. This means that in only 5 out of 100 or 1 out of 20 times would the outcome occur by chance. But in the Nurses' Health Study, the results were much more impressive. Based on this and other observational studies, researchers thought that hormone therapy reduced cardiovascular disease by between 35 and 50 percent, an extremely impressive figure.

Another general observation was that heart disease tends to affect women a full ten to fifteen years later than it does men. Since this period of time coincides with menopause, there was a presumption that estrogen had protected women when they were younger. There was evidence that estrogen had a beneficial effect on lipids and that it might have positive effects on coagulation and act as an antioxidant, binding up those damaging free radical chemicals. All of these actions would explain the lower rate of cardiovascular disease. So the findings seemed completely plausible. One expert stated that she had a "stack of paper inches thick" on how estrogen might favorably affect the cardiovascular system.

Randomized Controlled Trials

The results of the large observational studies caused many physicians and health care professionals to begin to prescribe estrogen and combined estrogen plus progestin for the prevention of heart disease. Prevention of heart disease was never an FDA-approved use of estrogen, however, since the gold standard test of that use of estrogen had yet to be completed. Estrogen was FDA-approved only for the treatment of menopausal symptoms.

It is generally agreed that the following factors are needed to conclude that any treatment is effective: First, the subjects need to be randomly assigned to a treatment or a control group. This is usually done with a system to generate random numbers, placing each subject in his or her assigned treatment group. Randomization, if it works, should make the two groups alike in all respects except the treatment. Second, the subjects should be unaware, or blinded, as to which group they are in. The experimenters should be blinded also—that is, not know which subject is in which group. This is called a double-blind study. Third, the measure should be as objective as possible. The subjects should ideally have the same expectations for their treatment. They should be followed over long periods of time. When all these conditions are met, the study is called a randomized controlled trial, or an RCT.

So many people were so persuaded by the initial observational studies that the makers of Premarin applied to the Federal Drug Administration to add another indication, prevention of heart disease, for this medication's use. For women who had not had hysterectomies, the study would need to be done using Prempro, the combination of conjugated equine estrogen plus a progestin to eliminate the added risk of uterine cancer with estrogen alone. Only in women who had undergone hysterectomies could estrogen be used alone.

The postmenopausal estrogen/progestin interventions trial, or PEPI trial, was initiated by the National Institutes of Health in 1987. It revealed that although hormone therapy reduced LDL, the "bad" cholesterol, it increased other fats in the blood, the triglycerides. So the next trial was begun in order to determine whether hormone therapy could prevent additional heart attacks in women who had already had them.

The first major randomized controlled trial to look at the hormone therapy/heart disease connection was the heart and estrogen/progestin replacement study (HERS). The 2,763 women in this study already had a diagnosis of cardiovascular disease. That is, they had had heart attacks or heart surgery, or had significant blocked coronary arteries. They were randomized to either a placebo group or a group in which they took estrogen and progestin (Prempro). In 1998, after a little more than four years of follow-up, no differences in overall heart disease were found between the treated and the placebo groups. In fact, to the surprise of the investigators, there was a suggestion of an early increase in cardiac events among women who were taking estrogen and progestin. At that time, some hoped that the early increase in cardiac events would be outweighed by a later benefit. This would have explained the discrepancy between these findings and those from the Nurses' Health Study and other observational studies. This was not the case, however. An extension of the trial to 6.8 years of follow-up failed to confirm any late benefit. Thus, the conclusion of this first randomized controlled trial was that hormone therapy should not be used to reduce coronary heart disease, at least in women who already had the disease.

But what about women who did *not* have heart disease? That's why the federally funded Women's Health Initiative was started in 1993. Many women were shocked that it took that long for this major study to be instigated. After all, millions of American women had been taking hormone therapy for decades. In fact, a 1995 telephone survey of households in the U.S. revealed that 37.6 percent of all menopausal women were taking hormone therapy. It had become clear that estrogen was the "flash blaster." It could virtually eliminate vasomotor symptoms such as hot flashes and night sweats. It could also prevent osteoporosis. Still, there were many unanswered questions. Did estrogen have a protective effect on the heart in healthy women? Could women suffer any ill effects from hormone therapy? Were some of the observational studies correct when they suggested an increased rate of breast cancer in long-term hormone users? The Women's Health Initiative was designed to answer these as well as other questions.

Funded by the National Institutes of Health, the Women's Health Initiative examined over 144,000 women in 40 sites all over the country. There are several parts of the study still ongoing. One randomized controlled trial randomly selected women to be on estrogen plus progestin, EPT (Prempro), or a placebo. The goal was to examine the risks and the benefits of the long-term use of estrogen plus progestin. This part of the study was stopped after an average of 5.2 years rather than the previously planned 8.5 years because the number of breast cancer cases and the overall number of adverse events in the estrogen and progestin group exceeded the predetermined level that would stop the study. The conclusion became clear: The health risks of the combined hormone therapy outweighed the benefits. Rather than confirming a protective effect on the heart, the trial revealed that there was an increased risk of heart events—mostly nonfatal heart attacks—in the estrogen plus progestin group. The rate of cardiovascular events for women receiving estrogen plus progestin was 29 percent higher than those receiving placebo (37 vs. 30 per 10,000 person-years).

One of the few remaining reasons to prescribe long-term hormone therapy was the hope that it would prevent dementia. One combined analysis of 10 observational studies of postmenopausal use of estrogen revealed a 29 percent decreased risk of dementia in those women using estrogen. The authors of this analysis acknowledged, however, that the results were not conclusive because the studies were not well-done randomized controlled trials. The Women's Health Initiative Memory Study, or WHIMS, was designed to examine the effect of combined EPT on the development of dementia and Alzheimer's disease. It included more than 4,500 women participating in the larger WHI who were 65 years old or older. The women were assigned to either the EPT or the placebo group and were thoroughly evaluated for cognitive changes. After an average of approximately 4 years of follow up, 40 women in the hormone group were diagnosed with dementia, as opposed to 21 in the placebo group. This was statistically significant. Thus, women in the combined hormone group, to the continued surprise of most researchers, were not less likely to develop dementia. In contrast, they had double the risk of those in the placebo group.

This study appeared in the *Journal of the American Medical Association* in May 2003. The same issue also had two other articles from the WHI results. One confirmed the increased rate of strokes suffered by women taking the combined estrogen and progestin regimen. The other examined more general cognitive functioning. In this study, contrary to predictions, the cognitive functioning of the women in the hormone therapy group was slightly *worse* than that of the women in the placebo group. Once again, the results of the randomized controlled trial left many people dumbfounded.

No conclusions can yet be drawn about the effects of estrogen alone, since that arm of the study is ongoing. All of this has reinforced the fact that a treatment or remedy that has shown positive anecdotal effects and observationl evidence may not be proven effective once carefully studied in a randomized controlled trial. Although observational studies may seem very convincing, in the absence of true controls, final conclusions cannot be made.

The Current Status of Estrogen and Hormone Therapy

So where does all of this leave us with regard to the use of hormone therapy? The dramatic response to the WHI results demonstrated the power of a large, well-done study. Many doctors who had prescribed hormone therapy for years in the honest belief that its benefits greatly outweighed the suspected or proven risks were described as turning on a dime. The professional organizations quickly issued new opinion statements about menopausal hormone therapy. The American College of Obstetrics and Gynecology and the North American Menopause Society recommended against hormone therapy for the prevention of heart disease and advised caution in the use of HT for prevention of osteoporosis, suggesting that alternative therapies be considered. The National Association of Women's Health Nurse Practitioners came to similar conclusions.

In 2002, the U.S. Preventative Services Task Force published their updated recommendation for the use of EPT to prevent chronic conditions. They concluded that "the harmful effects of estrogen and progestin are likely to exceed the chronic disease prevention benefits in most women." They went on to add that they "could not determine whether the benefits of unopposed estrogen outweigh the harms for women who have had a hysterectomy." Between July and October 2002, prescriptions for Premarin and Prempro, responsible for $2 *billion* of sales in 2002, dropped 40 percent.

What can we conclude about the use of hormone therapy based on these results? First, it is important to remember that the results thus far apply only to the use of EPT—that is, estrogen and progestin. Was the progestin, the MPA in Prempro, the culprit? The results for estrogen alone in women without a uterus are scheduled to be released in 2005. Second, the results pertain only to the use of EPT for prevention of conditions and not to the use of EPT for menopausal symptom control. Finally, it is true that only one type of estrogen and one type of progestin were used. Some have suggested that the results cannot be generalized to any other type of estrogen and progestin. Nevertheless, the FDA has concluded that the results do apply to all estrogens and progestins by issuing new cautions for all types of estrogen and progestin products. At this point, the burden of proof is on the manufacturers of those other products to prove they behave differently.

On January 8, 2003, the Food and Drug Administration issued a press release outlining new labeling for all postmenopausal hormone therapies. This new labeling highlights the increased risk of heart disease, stroke, and breast cancer. It goes further to recommend consideration of non-estrogen treatments for the prevention of osteoporosis. Doctors are advised to prescribe the lowest dose of estrogen for the shortest amount of time. The FDA acknowledges that postmenopausal hormone therapy will be used for moderate to severe menopausal symptoms. This dramatic change in labeling clearly relegates hormone therapy to the treatment of menopausal symptoms that are severe or nearly so.

The increased risks of breast cancer and blood clots were in the range expected from the big observational studies, like the Nurses' Health Study, and the small number of randomized controlled trials (PEPI, HERS). So while this was not great news, neither was it totally unexpected. On the other hand, the increased risk for stroke was unexpected, as was the big shocker, the *increased* (not decreased) risk of heart disease. Even though hormone therapy was shown to help prevent osteoporosis and colon cancer, these benefits paled in comparison to the newly established risks. In the end, it was the increased risk of heart disease that tipped the balance of risks and benefits away from the use of HT for prevention. Subsequent analyses of Women's Health Initiative data were also sobering. In an older subset of women, the combined hormone therapy led to an increased, not decreased, risk of developing dementia. To make matters worse, the breast cancers that developed in women on combined hormone therapy were slightly larger and more likely to have spread to the lymph nodes and other organs.

Could the pendulum swing back? It is unlikely that the combination of estrogen plus progestin will ever be viewed again as a magic bullet. Some physicians are challenging some of the results of the WHI. They point out that, while increases in breast cancer and heart disease were the negative outcomes, there were some positive effects, too, with a 37 percent reduction in colorectal cancer and 50 percent fewer fractures from osteoporosis. One author adds that 97.5 percent of the entire group of women in the WHI suffered no adverse event of any kind.

Another criticism of the WHI is the age of the subjects, with an average age of 63 and an age range of 50 to 79 years. Younger women with severe menopausal symptoms probably did not enroll in the study because they would not be willing to risk being randomized to a placebo group. Could it be that the further away you are from menopause, the less benefit you could derive from hormone therapy to prevent heart disease?

It is also important to remember that for any *individual woman*, the risks are still very small. Even though the percentage increases—26 percent in breast cancer; 29 percent in heart disease; 41 percent in strokes; and 100 percent in blood clots—sound terrifying, they are all fractional increases of small numbers. That is why the results are also reported as the increase or decrease in cases of a particular condition for every 10,000 person-years. This person-year number is the number of women taking HT multiplied by the number of years they remain on HT. So 10,000 person-years could be 2,000 women taking HT for five years, or 1,000 women taking HT for ten years, and so on.

Here is the breakdown if we express the change in outcomes for every 10,000 person-years of women on HT versus placebo:

- 7 *more* heart attacks (37 vs. 30)
- 8 *more* strokes (29 vs. 21)
- 8 *more* lung clots (16 vs. 8)
- 8 *more* breast cancers (38 vs. 30)

- 23 *more* cases of dementia for women 65 and older (45 vs. 22)
- 6 *fewer* colorectal cancers (10 vs. 16)
- 5 *fewer* hip fractures (10 vs. 15)

It is still difficult to wrap your mind around these statistics because they ultimately have meaning only when you consider a large population of women.

What do *we* think? Based on currently available information, we agree with the major women's health professional associations that:

- Hormone therapy should not be prescribed for the prevention of heart disease.
- Given the long-term risks, there are better alternatives for the prevention of osteoporosis.
- In contrast, the benefits of hormone therapy to treat moderate to severe hot flashes for a short term may well outweigh the risks. We will discuss this further in Chapter 3.
- Just as there was no "one size fits all" reason for every woman to take hormones before the Women's Health Initiative, there is no blanket rule to completely avoid them now. What is more important is to make an informed decision that is right for you.
- With so much research ongoing, don't make a decision everytime you read a headline in a newspaper. Your annual appointment with your primary care professional is the ideal time to reevaluate.

Taking these controversies as well as the rapid development of new products into consideration, we should learn the lessons of the past. When you hear about the results of a study or talk to a friend who believes in a certain treatment, you might ask the following questions:

- Is your source of information credible?
- Was the research done by expert researchers at a reputable institution?
- Was this study done on a large group of people or was it a smaller study? Was it an animal study? You will sometimes see the term *meta-analysis*. This is a statistical method that combines the results of several studies. It does so based on specific criteria, such as minimum number of subjects, use of

control groups, and a specifically defined outcome. The advantage of this technique is that it can utilize the information from well-done smaller studies rather than necessitating larger, often very expensive trials.

- Were the women in the study similar to you (in age, ethnicity, medical conditions, and so forth)?
- Were the patients randomized to treatment or placebo?
- Were the researchers and patients blind to the assignment of treatment or placebo?
- Did the study report any of the side effects of the treatment?
- Was the study conducted over an appropriate period of time? A study can report changes in a patient's current symptom in a few weeks or months. That's fine if you are going to take a medication for a short period of time, but as we've seen, it may take years for long-term consequences to be documented.
- Were the measurements used in the study objective?
- How significant was the effect of treatment? In other words, was the effect of treatment large enough that you would notice it?
- Was there complete follow-up of patients? If not, how many patients were lost to follow-up?
- Overall, was the treatment's benefit worth its potential harm?
- Who paid for the study?
- Do you see any evidence of bias? (If midlife women are referred to as "castrated" or "bovine," for example, you should stop reading.)
- Does the study mention whether the conclusion is consistent with previous research in the same area? If not, that probably means more research is needed and you shouldn't accept the results without further investigation.
- What is the perspective of other experts in the field? Many important studies are published with separate editorial comments written by experts.

These are just some of the questions you should ask yourself before jumping to conclusions. This doesn't mean you might not try a certain treatment anyway. However, you do need to make sure that the treatment is safe. We have mentioned this with respect to herbal preparations as opposed to those approved by the Federal Drug Administration. Some changes, such as those involving diet or modification of habits, are relatively free of side effects (as long as you agree that periodic hunger pains are not side effects!). You also need to know if any product interacts with any of your prescription and over-the-counter medications, so you should check with your physician and/or pharmacist. Also, think about the placebo effect and the financial cost. If placebos reduce hot flashes by up to a third, you might think long and hard before shelling out $19.99 for twenty tablets of anything that has only a slightly greater effect on your hot flashes.

Armed with this review of the research methods, you'll be better able to judge any studies or claims about the effectiveness of menopause treatments. In the chapters that follow, we will use some of these same analytical tools to review various treatment and prevention options.

CHAPTER THREE

Treating the Symptoms of Menopause

So much attention has been paid to hormone therapy that research on some of the other treatments for menopausal symptoms is relatively new. In the past, the options have usually been summarized as hormone therapy or "something else." It is true that there is a vast body of research about hormone therapy, so we know a lot. Nonetheless, there are numerous other options. One of the options, by the way, is *no* treatment. A symptom that may be troublesome to one woman may not even be noticed by another woman. Only you can know what needs to be treated.

Once again, here are the main symptoms of menopause: First, often beginning with perimenopause, hot flashes and night sweats occur, and may last for a few months or years. Later, a few years after the last menstrual cycle, vaginal dryness and other gynecological and urological symptoms may begin. These, along with changes in the menstrual cycle, are the only menopausal symptoms that professionals agree result from estrogen loss. Mood changes, memory, and quality of life issues are more complicated, and we will address these later in this chapter. There are other conditions associated with estrogen loss, but vasomotor, urinary, and gynecological symptoms are the most common. So please don't fall into the trap of blaming any and all symptoms on menopause.

Treatment of Hot Flashes

Hot flashes are associated with the decrease in estrogen levels. In fact, many women experience hot flashes after pregnancy, when estrogen levels go from very high back to normal. The decrease in estrogen, as we discussed in Chapter 1, disrupts the part of the brain that controls body temperature and the circulatory system. Amazingly, the precise cause of hot flashes is still not fully understood. After irregular periods, hot flashes and night sweats are the most common symptoms. They are referred to as vasomotor symptoms because they involve changes in the circulation, including increased temperature, heart rate, and blood flow.

Even though you might not know exactly *why* a hot flash occurs, you'll know when you have a severe one. Your skin temperature rises, your upper body feels hot and turns red, and you sweat profusely and then feel a chill. A few women feel only a chill. There is tremendous variability in women's experiences of hot flashes, but as many as 75 to 85 percent of perimenopausal women have them. Some women may feel a mild and even pleasant sensation of heat, and some may even be able to ignore them completely. Hot flashes tend to be worse when a woman has had her ovaries removed or has had menopause induced by medications such as chemotherapy.

About 15 percent of women experience severe hot flashes. The good news is that hot flashes ultimately will go away even without any treatment. The bad news is that it may take years. So you may or may not want to treat hot flashes based on how much they disrupt your life. If you are having severe, frequent hot flashes that interfere with your work or family life or are having night sweats that cause you to have insomnia, you may want to consider the following options.

Estrogen

Despite the many controversies about the use of estrogen, there is no doubt about its effectiveness in treating hot flashes. This makes perfect sense, since it is the loss of estrogen that presumably causes hot flashes. Estrogen therapy effectively controls hot flashes in more than 95 percent of women. Most women are treated with 0.625 milligrams of conjugated equine estrogen (Premarin) or its equivalent. Premarin is the oldest form of estrogen, but many others have been approved that are equally effective. Some women may require higher doses, whereas others may be treated with less. For control of symptoms, the general rule is to use the lowest estrogen dose that works. Recent studies document that lower doses of oral estrogen preparations, or about half of the usual dose for the treatment of hot flashes, can be effective in many women.

Unless you've had a hysterectomy, it is still necessary to add a progestin. This eliminates the potential increased risk of uterine (endometrial) cancer with estrogen alone. The duration of therapy depends on the duration of symptoms, but usually ranges from one to three years. Although most women experience hot flashes for fewer than five years after their last period, some may have them for up to ten years. (We wish it were otherwise, but there it is.) If you want to discontinue ET, it should be tapered off rather than stopped abruptly, as hot flashes may return with the sudden fall in estrogen levels.

Even though estrogen is the most effective treatment for hot flashes, it is by no means the only option. Given the risks of HT for any woman and especially for women with breast cancer, uterine cancer, and/or heart disease, these other therapies may be the best first choices for treatment of hot flashes. Placebos can reduce hot flash frequency by 20 to 30 percent, so some treatments are only marginally effective when considered against these fairly dramatic reductions. For new hot flash treatments, any promising anecdotal reports should be interpreted with great caution.

When we first met Jenny, she was a 52-year-old bookkeeper whose daughter was in junior college. Jenny's husband is a carpenter and she works part-time. She also enjoyed her small menagerie of three dogs and two cats. She had a shy but engaging manner. Like many patients, Jenny "didn't want to bother" us, but her hot flashes were "really annoying." We were actually quite relieved to hear the word *annoying* because we have heard a lot worse! Jenny's hot flashes were clearly disruptive, but not "hideously awful," "driving her crazy," or described through uncontrollable tears, as we have seen with some other patients. Jenny had read that estrogen was associated with breast cancer and did not protect against heart disease. Still, Jenny rated her hot flashes as detrimental to her sleep and troubling during the day. We explained to Jenny that estrogen therapy (combined with the necessary progestin) would still be the most effective treatment for her hot flashes. The increased risk of breast cancer was seen, on average, after four years of combined hormone therapy in the WHI participants. Even so, the breast cancers, when diagnosed, were at a later stage, making it imperative that Jenny use hormone therapy for the shortest time necessary. We warned her that an additional finding was that there was an increased rate of abnormal mammograms even after one year of treatment. Jenny decided to take hormone therapy for a few months and promised to be diligent about breast self-exams, breast exams performed by a physician, and yearly mammograms. Jenny was impressed by the quick elimination of her hot flashes.

If Jenny had been adamant about avoiding estrogen, we would also have respected her decision. Here are other options.

Behavioral Strategies

All women with hot flashes should use behavioral strategies because they are so straightforward. When used with a hot flash diary, such strategies can also help to provide a road map for future treatment. Behavioral strategies involve environmental planning and relaxation. Many women find it helpful to dress in layers of clothing. In addition, sleeping in a cool room can help. A hot flash diary can identify triggers, which may include specific foods (chocolate, for example), alcoholic drinks, caffeinated beverages, spicy or hot foods, and hot beverages. These triggers, once identified, can be avoided.

Relaxation and slow, deep abdominal breathing can reduce the severity of hot flashes. The relaxation response, or paced respirations, can be implemented at the beginning of a hot flash to stop or control it. The relaxation response is a technique that produces a change in your physiology. If you learn to relax, there will be a decrease in muscle tension and lowered blood pressure, as well as a decrease in heart rate and rate of breathing. Different ways to learn the relaxation response include progressive muscle relaxation, meditation, yoga, and prayer. Popular books include Dr. Herbert Benson's *The Relaxation Response* and

Dr. Joan Borysenko's *Inner Peace for Busy People: 52 Simple Strategies for Transforming Your Life*. There is also a CD, *Meditation for Optimum Health*, by Drs. Andrew Weil and Jon Kabat-Zinn. We'll give you more suggestions for ways to reduce stress in Chapter 4. One study revealed that women who learned the relaxation response showed a greater decrease in intensity and number of hot flashes and more improvement in depressed mood than a control group of women.

Exercise on a regular basis can help to minimize sleep disturbance. Exercise is also one of the best strategies to maintain health and improve mood. Small studies have found that twenty minutes of exercise each day can improve mood and may reduce the intensity of hot flashes. The best way to begin an exercise program depends on your level of fitness. If you haven't had any regular exercise recently, start out slowly, perhaps with walking. We will discuss the strategies of beginning and maintaining an exercise program in Chapter 4. Be sure to check in with your doctor before you begin any exercise program.

Herbal Therapies

Although herbal remedies may have promise as treatments for hot flashes, at the current time the buyer should beware. Since as previously mentioned, herbal preparations do not go through the levels of testing that the FDA requires for medications, the labeling and marketing of these remedies are virtually unregulated. We are often surprised by women who are totally skeptical of the medical establishment and pharmaceutical companies, yet naively accepting of claims for herbal therapies.

The following herbs have been promoted in the treatment of hot flashes and menopausal symptoms: black cohosh, cranberry, red clover, dong quai, evening primrose, ginseng, licorice, and sage. Most of these have not been studied by randomized controlled trials.

Black cohosh, also called snake root or bugbane, shows some promise. Black cohosh is a member of the buttercup family, a perennial plant native to North America with estrogen-like properties. The American College of Obstetricians and Gynecologists concluded that black cohosh may be helpful to treat hot flashes in the short-term (six months or less). The German Regulatory Authority, Commission E, also approves it for the treatment of menopausal symptoms. However, a study of women with breast cancer did not find black cohosh to be an effective treatment for hot flashes. This result may be explained by the fact that almost all of the women were taking the medication tamoxifen, known to intensify hot flashes. Tamoxifen also acts as an anti-estrogen and may block some of the estrogen-like effects of black cohosh.

A small study of German women compared black cohosh to combined HT and to placebo for three months. Both HT and black cohosh reduced hot flashes more than placebo. In addition, after three months, black cohosh did not lead to a thickening of the uterine lining. So black cohosh shows some effectiveness. Since black cohosh contains phytoestrogens, its safety for use by women with breast cancer is questionable.

Other trials of herbal remedies have been less promising. Dong quai, when studied, was no better than a placebo. It is known that women on blood-thinning medications also should not take it. Red clover was studied in two small clinical trials in Australia, but after three months was found to offer no significant benefit. One study of ginseng found it no better than placebo for treating menopausal symptoms, but did find a positive effect on mood. There have been reports of postmenopausal bleeding after the use of ginseng, so once again, safety is a concern. In another study, evening primrose had no effect on hot flashes.

If you are interested in herbal medications, Drs. Fredi Kronenberg and Adriane Fugh-Berman thoroughly reviewed all the randomized controlled trials of herbal treatments. They concluded that only black cohosh was documented to be more effective than placebo in treating hot flashes. Still, they added that the long-term safety of black cohosh has not been proven. There is a concern that black cohosh's estrogen-like properties may cause stimulation of breast and endometrial tissue. Its safety for women with breast cancer and uterine cancer has not been proven. Talk with your health care professional about any herbal preparations, and stay tuned, armed with your knowledge about research. You might visit the Web site of the National Center for Complementary and Alternative Medicine, part of the National Institutes of Health, at www.nccam.nih.gov, which can keep you up-to-date on new research with herbal therapies and new clinical trials. The Resources section at the back of the book will give you additional ways to find out about helpful treatments.

Vitamin E

The safety of vitamin E in low doses—800 international units (IU) a day or less—makes it a very reasonable first-line treatment. Until recently, most of the data on vitamin E was based on small reports. One trial of 800 IU per day of vitamin E compared it to a placebo in breast cancer survivors. The authors found only a marginal reduction in hot flash frequency, with only one less hot flash a day on average. But any individual woman may have a more dramatic response. Since vitamin E may very well have a benefit in preventing heart disease and has not been shown to have toxicity or side effects at the appropriate dosage, it is a good choice. For these reasons Drs. Walter Willett and Meir J. Stampfer of Harvard Medical School conclude that vitamin E supplements are appropriate for a middle-aged woman because the potential benefits outweigh the harms.

If none of these treatments works well for you, there are others. Quite a few medications that are not derived from estrogen can be helpful in the treatment of hot flashes. Of course, you will need to discuss these options with your primary care professional.

Clonidine

Clonidine (Catapres) is a medication used to treat high blood pressure. There is some evidence that clonidine can reduce hot flashes, but its use is often limited by side effects, including dry mouth, fatigue, and dizziness. Still, if these side effects are not distressing, clonidine may be a reasonable choice, especially if you also have high blood pressure.

Progestins

Different types of progestins have been effective. One form, medroxyprogesterone acetate (MPA, or Provera), is a pill. One study found that 10 to 20 milligrams twice a day led to a drop in the frequency of hot flashes by 90 percent. Megestrol acetate (Megace) is another type of progestin that has been used to treat metastatic breast cancer. Low doses of megestrol acetate (20 milligrams twice a day) have been shown to reduce hot flashes by 50 percent compared to a 20 percent reduction with placebo. However, more than half the women developed uterine bleeding. Some women experience side effects of depressed mood and weight gain, so the use of megestrol acetate should be monitored. This treatment could have special promise for women with breast cancer if its long-term safety is established. Since it is not known whether megestrol acetate affects hormonally sensitive cancers such as breast and uterine cancer, it cannot be recommended at this time with complete confidence as an alternative to estrogen for hot flashes.

Antidepressants

More recently, antidepressants have been studied for their effect on hot flashes. Promising results for venlafaxine (Effexor) have been published, with a dose of 75 milligrams a day, reducing hot flash frequency by 60 percent among breast cancer survivors. A pilot trial of paroxetine (Paxil), starting with 10 milligrams a day and increasing to 20 milligrams a day, has shown promising results as well, with a 67 percent reduction in hot flash frequency. There was no control group. Fluoxetine (Prozac) has also been shown to reduce hot flashes but is somewhat less effective than venlafaxine. Since depressed mood is another common symptom in women, these results are particularly promising for women experiencing depression as well as hot flashes.

And Keep Your Eye on Progesterone Cream

There is currently a lot of interest in progesterone cream used alone, without estrogen, to treat hot flashes. In the United States, progesterone cream is sold over-the-counter as Pro-Gest, containing 20 milligrams progesterone per teaspoon, or 450 milligrams per ounce. In one small trial, 87 percent of women found that 450 milligrams of Pro-Gest cream was effective in treatment of hot flashes, compared to 19 percent of those in the placebo group. However, a larger Australian study of 32 milligrams daily for twelve weeks did not find changes in hot flashes, mood, sexual feelings, lipid levels, or bone. In addition, the absorption of transdermal progesterone cream varies from woman to woman. More research is needed before we jump on this bandwagon.

A lot of advertising promotes wild yam cream as containing "precursors to progesterone." But guess what? Experts suggest that it is unlikely to be converted to progesterone within the body. Other advertising promotes creams made up of both wild yam cream and progesterone produced in a lab. Confused? Skeptical? We are. Thus far, claims for wild yam creams have not been substantiated.

Soy Products

Interest in soy protein as a treatment for menopausal symptoms began with the observation that Asian women report fewer hot flashes and have a diet high in soy protein. Soy protein contains phytoestrogen, or the isolated isoflavones genestein and daidzein, which have some estrogen-like properties. Most studies of soy have not shown significant reductions in hot flashes when compared to placebo. One study compared women eating soy flour to those eating wheat flour and found a placebo effect (wheat flour) of 25 percent, whereas the soy flour group had a 40 percent reduction in hot flashes. In another clinical trial of soy extract with breast cancer survivors, there was no demonstrated benefit from 50 milligrams a day versus placebo.

Soy Protein Content of Common Foods

FOOD	SOY PROTEIN (IN GRAMS)
Four ounces of firm tofu	13
One soy sausage link	6
One soy burger	10–12
One 8 ounce glass of plain soy milk	10
One soy protein bar	14
One-half cup of tempeh	19.5
1/4 cup roasted soy nuts	19
Soy sauce	0

Source: Adapted from FDA Consumer, 2003.

At this point, soy protein cannot be recommended as a very effective treatment for vasomotor symptoms. Research is ongoing, however, and the FDA has also suggested that 25 grams of soy protein is beneficial for heart health. Since soy has estrogen-like properties, soy supplements are not advisable for women with breast cancer. Remember that soy products are not monitored for the amount of active ingredients or purity, so read the labels and choose a reputable source.

Anticonvulsants

A promising medication in the treatment of hot flashes and night sweats is gabapentin (Neurontin). It was first noted to be beneficial for hot flashes based on the experience of six patients treated with the drug for other conditions. Hot flashes were reduced by 75 percent in these patients. A larger study revealed less impressive results but still found about a 50 percent reduction in frequency and severity, compared to about 30 percent with placebo. Additional studies are under way to confirm these very preliminary results.

Tibolone

Tibolone is a synthetic hormone with properties similar to estrogen, progestin, and testosterone. It is available in Europe, but not yet in Canada or the United States. It is used primarily to prevent osteoporosis, but has also been shown to be effective in reducing hot flashes. A Swedish study randomly assigned women to an estrogen-progesterone (EPT) combination or to tibolone. Tibolone was found to be as effective as the HT combination, but did not lead to as much vaginal bleeding.

Veralapride

Veralapride is a medication that affects brain chemistry, a neurotransmitter that now is available only in Europe. Studies suggest that it may be effective in treating hot flashes.

Acupuncture

Acupuncture is an ancient treatment, more recently applied as a treatment for hot flashes. Very thin sterile needles (they don't hurt, really!) are applied to various body points according to traditional Chinese medicine. It is established as an effective treatment for pain and as somewhat effective in the treatment of nausea in adults after chemotherapy and during pregnancy. In their review, however, Kronenberg and Fugh-Berman reported on only one small study of acupuncture as a treatment for hot flashes. In that study, there were no differences between women treated with acupuncture and those in the control group.

So there is a wide range of treatments for hot flashes, with more being developed every day. Be sure to enlist the help of your primary health care professional in making a safe choice. Don't forget to use your diary to monitor your progress.

Treatments for Sexual Functioning and Urinary Symptoms

Other symptoms due to estrogen loss are related to sexual functioning and the urinary tract. These problems include vaginal dryness, painful intercourse, painful urination, urinary incontinence, and urinary tract infections.

"I would really prefer not to talk about this, but . . ." This was the beginning of our conversation with Molly, a 58-year-old grandmother. "Yes, *grandmother* is how I like to think of myself," Molly told us. A widow for seven years, Molly was an energetic woman with a mop of strawberry-blond curls ("helped along by Clairol, and why not?"). She was then living on a decent pension and helping her three children with their five children, ages 4 to 11. We first saw Molly a few years ago. She was a pre-baby-boomer-generation woman and was extremely embarrassed to talk about her problems "down there." Since you, too, may be embarrassed, let us arm you with some information.

Here's what happens: As estrogen declines over time, two sets of changes occur. First there are changes in the structure of the gynecological and urinary, or pelvic, organs. The lining of the vaginal wall becomes thinner after menopause, with many fewer layers of cells. This is called vaginal atrophy. Thus, irritation, called vaginitis, can occur much more often. In addition, the vagina becomes shorter and narrower.

Sexual responses change a bit, too. The stages of sexual responses include excitement or arousal, plateau, orgasm, and resolution. During the arousal stage, the vagina becomes lubricated and muscle tension increases. After menopause, it takes longer for women to become aroused. In addition, some women report that the experience of orgasm is less intense. Unlike hot flashes, which get better over time, gynecological problems can get worse. They usually become noticeable some years after menopause if no treatment has occurred.

Two thirds of women are not particularly bothered by these changes, but there are a number of options for Molly and other women who do have difficulties. Even though Molly was not involved sexually, she experienced discomfort and worried that this would interfere with future relationships. She felt periodic burning, and her pelvic exam was painful when the doctor tried to insert the speculum. Molly told us about her bothersome vaginal dryness ("it is itchy at times").

We explained to Molly that symptoms of burning and itching may be caused by a number of urinary or gynecological conditions. Urinary tract infections may cause burning at the time of urination and frequent urges to urinate. Vaginal infections, including yeast infections, may also cause burning because of inflammation around the vagina, and may be accompanied by a vaginal discharge. Sometimes menopausal changes in the vagina can cause some of these symptoms. To sort this out, a pelvic examination and urinalysis are necessary.

We shared some of the treatment possibilities.

Estrogen

Since these vaginal symptoms are results of estrogen decline, they can be treated quite effectively with estrogen. In this situation, topical estrogen, in the form of vaginal tablets, rings, or creams, can be used. These are more effective than pills by mouth or patches for the gynecological symptoms because they provide more estrogen where it is needed. The doses vary depending on the type of cream or tablet used.

There are different ways that vaginal estrogen might be prescribed. One strategy is daily use for three weeks and then twice a week thereafter. A 25-microgram tablet containing estradiol (Vagifem) is available in the United States and is inserted into the vagina twice weekly. A lower dose (10 micrograms) is available in Europe. With low-dose vaginal estrogens, progestin is not usually prescribed. Some women who are using high-dose estrogen do need to add a progestin.

A vaginal ring, Estring, can be placed in the vagina, releasing estrogen continuously in small amounts for three months. The advantage is that there is less absorption into the bloodstream than with other vaginal estrogens. One study found that women preferred the vaginal ring to vaginal creams.

Moisturizers and Lubricants

There are several alternative treatments as well. Conventional moisturizers can be helpful. At first Molly told us that she did not have a partner, so she was not concerned about intercourse. Some women who have vaginal dryness develop pain during intercourse, or dyspareunia. In this situation, a water-based lubricant, like Astroglide, can be helpful. A longer-lasting moisturizer, including Replens or KY Long-Lasting Vaginal Moisturizer, can be used three times a week. These are nonhormonal bioadhesive moisturizers. Oil-based products, such as Vaseline, should be avoided because they cause irritation and also allow bacteria to cling to the vaginal wall. Moisturizers may take up to four weeks to increase vaginal lubrication and up to twelve weeks to increase vaginal elasticity.

Molly's case points out that not all burning and itching is a yeast infection. Therefore, some women think that douching will remove their symptoms. Bad idea. Douching can make things worse by disrupting the vaginal ecosystem.

Treatment and Prevention
of Urinary Symptoms

Similar to the changes in the gynecological organs, the urethra, or the canal that carries urine from the bladder out of the body, becomes shorter. This allows bacteria to get into the bladder more easily and infection can occur. The standard treatment for a urinary tract infection (UTI) is an antibiotic.

It is also wise to avoid future UTIs, so several behavioral and hygiene strategies can help. First, drink lots of fluids to flush out the urinary tract. Cranberry juice, an old-fashioned cure that changes the pH, or acidity, of the urine, can be helpful. Cotton underwear is better than synthetic, since it does not hold in heat and moisture. Be careful about wiping yourself from front to back after a bowel movement to avoid spreading bacteria.

Incontinence

For Molly, incontinence was not a major problem: "It happens now and then, not a big deal." It did not interfere with her daily activities. But Molly was concerned about her future: "I don't want to end up like poor June Allyson in those awful old commercials!" We understood her reluctance, since incontinence is still a bit of a taboo topic. Yet more women are becoming aware of it because protective shields are now routinely advertised on prime-time television. Unfortunately, the message in these ads is that the problem is unique to elderly women. Not true. In fact, 30 percent of midlife women have this problem, but fewer than half of them seek help. For Molly and most women, this is still an embarrassing symptom to discuss, and some women even believe that it is inevitable and untreatable.

Basically, incontinence is the involuntary loss of urine and is classified into two major types. Molly had experienced periodic stress incontinence, the loss of urine that occurs with anything that can increase pressure on the bladder, including laughing, coughing, or bearing down to lift something. This type of incontinence tends to get worse with age unless preventive measures are taken. The cause of stress incontinence is the weakening and relaxation of the muscles and ligaments holding the pelvic organs in place. Like any muscle or ligament, these can weaken over time unless strengthened with exercise. It is also true that estrogen maintains their elasticity and strength. Women who are most prone to this type of incontinence are those who have had multiple pregnancies that can stretch and weaken some of the connecting structures of the pelvic organs.

The second, less common type of incontinence is urge incontinence. This is experienced as an inability to hold the urine whenever there is the urge to urinate. Women who have experienced this type of incontinence need to urinate immediately. Urge incontinence seems to be related to a weakening of the specific muscle that controls urination. For some women, this can be a major problem. In these cases, a complete evaluation is warranted. This could include urine cultures, studies of the bladder function, and a complete gynecological exam. There are effective medications available, and in some cases, surgery may be the best choice.

Kegel Exercises

Pelvic-floor exercises, or Kegel exercises, can increase the blood circulation to the pelvic floor and decrease the likelihood of urinary incontinence. Developed by a surgeon, Dr. Arnold Kegel, in the 1950s, these exercises increase muscle tone. They involve tensing and relaxing the pubococcygeal muscles, those around the area of the urethra and vagina. In order to identify these muscles, you can begin to urinate and then stop. The same muscle you use to control urination is the muscle that you will contract and relax during Kegel exercises. You can also locate and use this muscle by inserting a tampon and squeezing around it. You should hold this muscle for at least five to ten seconds and release it slowly. Then after mastering the slow Kegel exercise, you should also do a series of rapid ones. They should be repeated 10 to 15 times, and the whole session should be repeated three to five times per day. Between 50 and 70 percent of women with incontinence improve by performing Kegel exercises often. Actually, you can do them anywhere, anytime you feel like it. If you have difficulty doing the pelvic-floor exercises, some doctors and physical therapists specialize in this area of women's health care. A few urologists and/or gynecologists specialize in incontinence and can make a referral to a physical therapist.

Sexuality

As a woman gets to know her doctor better, she becomes increasingly open about problems. Sometimes the presenting complaint is not always the only, or certainly the most important, one. As time went by, we learned more about Molly and she revealed additional details of her sexual life and concerns. Her vaginal symptoms had been successfully treated and we'd given her some ideas to prevent future problems. We also hoped that by doing Kegel exercises, she could prevent the development of incontinence. Molly was now comfortable discussing these once-taboo topics. And so it came up that although Molly was not sexually involved at the moment, neither had she completely retired. When we mentioned that Kegel exercises were helpful to prevent incontinence and also to improve sexual functioning, Molly opened up. She had attended Al-Anon for several years because her late husband had been a recovering alcoholic. Recently she had run into a man, Ken, at the grocery store, whom she had met years before at a meeting. He, too, was widowed. Molly had some future plans for this man but wondered if she could become sexually active again after all these years.

This can be a difficult situation for women who develop vaginal thinning after menopause and don't have any treatment. But the same treatments we suggested thus far—moisturizers, Kegel exercises—could help Molly "get back in shape." Molly could also have chosen a short course of vaginal estrogen therapy. This could treat the vaginal dryness and the thinning. And for the short-term treatment of symptoms, there are fewer risks of estrogen therapy. When estrogen is used vaginally, this typically results in very low blood levels of estrogen. Molly promised that she would tell us the results of her new love interest.

For other women, too, it is critically important to assess the precise nature of the problem. Molly's problems were pain and itching. Other women may have problems with a lack of sexual interest, or libido. Still others may have problems with sexual arousal. By the way, here is another good reason to exercise—it may well facilitate sexual arousal. One study found that women who exercised on a stationary bike were more aroused by an erotic movie than those who didn't. And women who exercise regularly feel more self-confident about their bodies.

All of the sexual problems can occur at the same time. It is helpful to be very clear as to the nature of your sexual concerns and issues with your primary care professional. He or she can help you sort this out. For example, pain during sexual intercourse would naturally lead to an avoidance of sexual behavior. This can be treated, as we have discussed. On the other hand, a decrease in sexual interest or desire can be a result of many other factors, including stress, fatigue, and depression. Moreover, several of the antidepressant medications have the side effect of a decreased libido and lack of orgasm. Some of the commonly prescribed antidepressants are fluoxetine (Prozac), paroxetine (Paxil), sertraline (Zoloft), and citalopram (Celexa). (You can change medications or add another in order to deal with this side effect. Talk to your doctor.) So you can see why a full discussion and evaluation is a good idea.

Now let's put midlife sexuality in a larger context. One of the advantages of getting older should be increased leisure time and less self-consciousness. This combination can allow for greater sexual freedom. For example, if a woman has difficulty with arousal, then more time should be spent on oral or manual stimulation. Sensuality, or greater awareness of body pleasure in general, can enhance sexual functioning. Masturbation is always an option. For those women in long-term relationships, changing the romantic and sexual routines can rekindle interest and arousal.

Remember, too, that the sexual organs respond well to practice. Continued sexual activity prevents some of the postmenopausal changes by mucosal stimulation. This has been referred to as the "use it or lose it" principle. For women who have established symptoms of vaginal atrophy, a short course of vaginal estrogen may be helpful at first.

"Use it or lose it" may be more difficult than it sounds, especially if a couple has never discussed sexuality. The couple needs to begin with as honest a conversation as possible. Concerns and desires should be discussed in a nonjudgmental fashion. Communication, experimentation, and relaxation are three key elements. With respect to relaxation, allow more time for sex. A bath or massage can help set the stage for a relaxed sexual experience. Experimentation can involve fantasies, erotic materials, and oral, manual, or vibrator stimulation.

But none of this will occur without good communication. Intimacy and sensuality are inextricably linked, especially for women. And intimacy requires openness, verbal and nonverbal communication, even about complex and somewhat difficult subjects like sexual function and sexual dysfunction. This can become more anxiety provoking because guess what? Midlife and older men also have lots of sexual problems and concerns. In fact, a study of midlife Australian women found that women's sexuality was affected by two primary factors. These were the women's emotional attachment to their partners and the sexual difficulties of the partners, not of the women themselves. Men may also have sexual dysfunction as a side effect of several common types of medications, including those for high blood pressure and, once again, the antidepressants. In addition, men may have problems with erectile dysfunction as they grow older, especially if they have diabetes or heart disease. Many women are afraid of hurting their partner's egos by bringing up erectile difficulties. But in a noncritical, mutual discussion, the subject can be explored sensitively. So let's not take all the responsibility for midlife sexual dysfunction. This, too, can be shared.

In our work with lesbian women, we find that communication is different, but can be subject to similar stresses as in heterosexual couples. Research on menopausal lesbian couples is scarce. Lesbians have, obviously, the shared understanding of female sexuality. In addition, it has been suggested that lesbian women are more satisfied sexually than heterosexual women. However, if there is an age difference, the woman who reaches midlife and menopause first will need to be open about her sexual changes and needs. And if the couple does not have the ability to communicate about potential sexual problems, stresses can develop. Some of our patients also joke about "lesbian bed death," a condition in which the couple in a long-term relationship is contented, but not involved sexually to a great degree. This can happen to heterosexual couples as well and is not necessarily a problem when both partners feel comfortable.

Some women are saddened by the lack of a partner. This may be especially annoying to midlife heterosexual women when they watch 60-something men date 30-something women (think Michael Douglas and Catherine Zeta-Jones, or Harrison Ford and Calista Flockhart). Nevertheless, there are still a few reasonable older men left, as well as newer, less humiliating singles groups, like Singles Who Volunteer, which combine social activities with projects such as working for Habitat for Humanity.

Sexual Dysfunction

Sometimes a woman or a couple has more serious sexual difficulties. These may be a result of more general relationship problems or of a specific sexual dysfunction. In addition, if a woman has a history of sexual abuse, a change in sexual functioning can trigger psychological reactions. Individual therapy, couples therapy, or specific sex therapy can be helpful.

Try to be as open as possible, not only with your partner but with your doctor or primary care professional. Sexuality and urinary functions are still difficult to talk about. But as Molly revealed more, she was able to learn more as well. So, Molly could take better care of herself and enjoy her sexual future.

And Keep Your Eye on Testosterone

Changes in sexual desire and decreased sexual responsiveness may be completely separate from any vaginal symptoms. Sometimes the vaginal symptoms are treated first only to reveal that the real problem is an independent loss of libido. If other possible contributory factors have been ruled out, some physicians will consider prescribing testosterone, even though it is not FDA-approved for this purpose. Most of the small number of studies in which testosterone has been shown to increase sex drive have involved women whose ovaries have been removed.

Estratest, a combination of estrogen and testosterone, is FDA-approved for treatment of hot flashes that do not respond to estrogen alone. However, doctors have prescribed it for treating a decrease in libido in perimenopausal or menopausal women.

Still, testosterone products are in development. Before considering testosterone, you'll need to weigh the substantial risks against the potential benefits. These include elevated cholesterol, liver function abnormalities, and masculinization (hirsutism, acne, lowering of the voice, and clitoral enlargement). Furthermore, there are no long-term studies of the effects of testosterone on women.

Viagra and Other Remedies

There are ongoing trials of sildenafil, Viagra, to see if it improves sexual response in women. Early studies of women did not find such effects at doses of 10, 50, or 100 milligrams. In addition, the higher doses were associated with headache and flushing at rates higher than those found in men.

Recently we've noticed TV and magazine ads for Avlimil, which is touted to be the cure-all for female sexual dysfunction. We checked it out to see if the ads had any scientific validity. According to their Web site, Avlimil is a nonprescription, "nonsynthetic, nonhormonal, and proven effective" treatment to improve and enhance sexual functioning in women. The medication includes a "proprietory blend of herbs," the major component of which is *Salvia officinalis*, or sage. However, there are no clinical trials published in peer-reviewed medical journals as of this date. Did we say this before? Buyer beware.

It's worth repeating: Sex is all about feeling good about yourself, open communication, and sharing. You have so many choices. Experiment and relax if you do have a partner; if you don't have a partner, you can still experiment and relax. If you're not overly sexual, be romantic and/or sensual. Try to focus on pleasure, not necessarily orgasm. If you have some problems, talk to your partner so you can work on sex together. Talk to your doctor as well, so that you can learn more about treatment choices. And remember that another key sexual organ is the brain. Try to keep your attitude positive. Not a Pollyannaish or rose-colored-glasses attitude, but a mature, humorous, and open one. Check out the Resources at the end of the book. It might also help you to know that the name of one of the menopause support groups is called the Red Hot Mamas.

Quality of Life, Mood, and Memory

Hot flashes, as well as sexual/urinary problems, are the primary symptoms associated with menopause. We are including this section on mood problems, quality of life, and memory because so many women ask about

them at our public seminars. Unlike hot flashes and the sexual and urinary changes, mood problems are not seen as directly related to the hormonal changes of menopause. So if you are just entering perimenopause
or the menopause transition, don't believe that you're about to crash.
That's one of the myths we debunked in Chapter 1. Most women manage their moods quite well. In fact, a Gallup Poll taken in 1998 revealed
that most women felt happier than ever before. Still, there are some
groups of women who may be more vulnerable to mood problems.

Although natural menopause does not lead to clinical depression in
most women, some women do experience depressed mood during this
time of life. Each woman's situation needs to be examined individually.
The best long-term studies of mood and menopause found that the
women most likely to become clinically depressed are those with significant family or health problems, not hormonal changes. In these situations cognitive behavior therapy, family counseling, and careful
management of medical problems are key elements of treatment. Antidepressant medication is also very effective.

Mood swings, or rapid changes in moods from irritability to tearful-
ness, normal to bad, may occur in perimenopausal, not postmenopausal,
women. They generally occur in about 10 percent of women. We sometimes hear women say "It's just like PMS—only worse." For most women,
these swings are time-limited.

A more persistent depressed mood, when a woman feels consistently
sad or edgy, is often associated with hot flashes. Several studies that followed women over time, or longitudinally, tell us a lot about mood
changes. The Massachusetts Women's Health Study, the Healthy Women
Study in Pittsburgh, and the Seattle Midlife Women's Health Study produced many helpful insights. Hot flashes and night sweats have been
implicated in causing depressed mood, especially when they go untreated
for long periods of time. Marcia, one of our clients, was able to describe
her depressed mood. "Every night I wake up sweating five or six times.
Pretty soon I'd start worrying about whether I would sleep. Then when I'd
wake up, I'd start worrying about not getting back to sleep. Then I'd keep
on worrying. During the day I feel like I can just barely get by. I'm usually
strong, but now the littlest thing gets to me. I feel nervous *and* sad."

Most experts agree that night sweats are causing Marcia's problems. Some have suggested that the hormonal changes disrupt sleep in-

dependent of night sweats. Marcia had several choices. She could try to tough it out, but we thought she had already suffered quite a bit.

Estrogen therapy has been shown to have some positive effect on mood changes, especially if they are associated with night sweats and hot flashes or are a result of surgical menopause. A recent large analysis of research concluded that estrogen therapy helps stabilize mood changes, but only in women with prominent hot flashes and night sweats. Estrogen also improves mood in women after surgical rather than natural menopause. Yet combination estrogen plus progestin therapy (EPT) causes some women to experience more depressed moods in response to progestins. In this situation, different forms of progestin may be tried, in the lowest possible doses. In Marcia's case, she went on EPT for six months. When she tapered off, she had a few night sweats, but many fewer now that the cycle of waking up and worrying was broken.

An actual clinical depressive episode is not a typical reaction to menopause. Since depression is so common in women, however, it can be difficult to sort out. Women become depressed two to three times more often than men, and approximately 25 percent of all women will have a major depressive episode in their lifetime. And most depressed people receive little or no treatment.

A major depressive episode occurs when you have a change in the way you think, act, and feel that lasts more than two weeks. If you have several of the following symptoms, you may well be clinically depressed:

- Depressed mood or a lack of interest in daily activities most of the day
- Changes in weight, sleeping, and physical activity
- A loss of energy and concentration
- Feelings of guilt or worthlessness
- Suicidal thoughts or thoughts of death

If you feel that you are this depressed or your family and friends think you are, please don't accept it as a normal symptom of menopause, but talk to your health care professional or go to a mental health professional (see the Resources). Psychotherapy and/or antidepressant medication can be extremely helpful. The SSRIs, or selective serotonin reuptake inhibitors, increase the available amount of serotonin, a neurotransmitter that helps improve mood. Older types of antidepressants (amitriptyline, or Elavil, for example) are equally effective in treating depression but produce more troubling side effects.

Herbal Treatment of Mood

Since anxiety and depression are the two most common psychological complaints of menopausal women, the two herbs taken most commonly are St. John's wort, used to improve mood, and valerian, used to decrease nervousness and insomnia. Both are approved and prescribed in Germany.

St. John's wort, or *Hypericum perforatum*, is a plant with a yellow flower that blooms in June, near St. John's Day. The Cochrane Group examined twenty-seven studies of the use of St. John's wort to treat mild to moderate depression. They concluded that the herb is superior to placebo, with fewer side effects than antidepressants. The usual dose is 300 milligrams (standardized to contain 5 percent hyperforin, 0.3 percent hypericin, or both) three times a day. It can take two to four weeks to work.

These studies, however, deal with mild to moderate *symptoms* of depressed mood, not a major depressive episode. There are studies in progress, but none yet has found St. John's wort to be superior to the SSRIs in treating a major depressive episode. One study found that it was not effective.

It's a good idea to take St. John's wort with food to minimize gastrointestinal side effects. Since this herb can also increase sensitivity to sunlight, it's important to wear sunscreen and a hat. St. John's wort should not be taken with another antidepressant. It can also interact with other medications, so a physician should be consulted.

Valerian, or *Valeriana officinalis*, is made from the roots of the plant and is used to decrease anxiety and promote sleep. While fewer studies have been done on valerian than on St. John's wort, controlled trials indicate that it is effective in promoting sleep. Reported long-term side effects include headache, restlessness, and cardiac disorders.

Quality of Life

What about quality of life or a general feeling of well-being? It is true that some women state that they just feel better taking estrogen. We feel that it is more helpful to target what the estrogen is actually treating. Hot flashes? Night sweats? Sleep? Otherwise, you could be experiencing a placebo effect and the risks would certainly outweigh the benefit. Research is ongoing to look at quality-of-life issues with more precision.

Memory

"What is her name? I know it . . . just wait." Memory, or the ability to take in and recall new information, declines a bit with aging in both women and men. Insomnia, stress, mood, and substance abuse can affect memory, and that's just a partial list. A large review of the literature found that hormones do affect neurotransmitters and brain functioning.

Memory problems can be more severe in cases of menopause induced by surgery and chemotherapy. Short-term studies of women who had their ovaries removed found that ET may help specifically with verbal memory. The emphasis here is on short-term relief and these results do not imply long-term benefits or protective effects.

For the average woman, the best general strategy is to keep an active cognitive life. Just as you exercise your body, you can keep your brain active with reading, crossword puzzles, and education. Some believe that the problem comes in how your brain stores the information. So, when you're 20 and you meet Rose, you remember her name. But when you're 50, you may need to say to yourself, "Rose. She has a flower's name." This helps you recall better because you've made an association. (Yes, you might end up calling her Iris, but this is a start.) Another tip: If you can't remember a name or you're not sure whether you've met someone, say "It's good to see you," not "It's good to see you again" or "Nice to meet you." Nudge your companion and hope he or she remembers.

Coping with New Information

Medical knowledge is exploding. We have found it challenging to summarize even the most recent studies on the treatment of menopausal symptoms. So we know that you will continue to face new headlines and quotes about the latest report on menopause long after you've finished this book. What is the best way to cope with forthcoming research? Here are some ideas.

- Review the terms and concepts we covered in Chapter 2 on women's health research. That way you'll know how seriously to take any new data.
- Look at the larger body of material. Does this study fit well into what we know already? Or does it take us in a new direction? If so, is it a large, well-controlled study that merits attention? If not, don't be hasty and accept uncritically any radical "new" results.
- Subscribe to a top-notch newsletter and/or Web site. We've listed several in the Resources at the end of this book, but the *Harvard Women's Health Watch* is one of the best. The views of its editorial board help put the news in context.
- In addition, certain journalists and specific general periodicals are reliable and current. Jane Brody and Gina Kolata at the *New York Times* and Judy Foreman of the *Boston Globe* come to mind. *Consumer Reports* often has excellent medical reviews. *Prevention*, a well-known magazine, is a good resource for news about exercise.
- The National Institute of Health Web site on women's health is excellent. If you don't have a computer, most public libraries have Internet access and staff available to help you. Many journal articles can be ordered from your local library or the National Library of Medicine, online at http://www.nlm.nih.gov.

How do we make sense of all this research on treatment choices? First, remember your priorities in terms of treating symptoms and current and future health goals. Once again, not every symptom requires treatment. You may not be bothered by a few hot flashes. We need to stop thinking that we can or should medicalize every experience associated with menopause. Other principles to keep in mind:

- Consider your comfort level with any increased risk of a bad outcome. For example, you know that taking hormone therapy over time increases your risk of breast cancer by 26 percent. But you know that this 26 percent increase still translates into a relatively low personal risk of getting breast cancer. Based on your psychological reactions to this risk, you may decide to choose hormone therapy or not.
- How comfortable are you with conducting a clinical experiment on yourself? In fact, a lot of clinical medicine is based on trial and error. Your willingness to experiment may depend on how much any symptom is disrupting your life or how much any preventable condition could affect you.
- The newer the treatment, the greater the degree of uncertainty. Any new medication or herbal therapy has not been studied long enough to ascertain its long-term consequences or adverse effects. For example, while selective estrogen receptor modulators (SERMs) show promise in preventing and treating osteoporosis, we do not know what impact they might have on the risk of Alzheimer's disease and do not have complete data on their effect on heart disease. If this level of uncertainty unsettles you, you might turn to a plan with less risk, such as calcium and exercise.

Finally, remember that no decision is forever. You can take the time to reflect on your choices and make new ones if you wish. You can talk to your friends and family. Your goals, needs, and health concerns also change over time. There are Resources to help you keep up-to-date at the end of this book. And in Chapters 7 and 8 we'll see how several women thought through their choices during their menopausal years.

◯─◯─◯

CHAPTER FOUR

Strong Bones and Healthy Hearts:

Preventing Osteoporosis and Heart Disease

As we grow older, we all want to maintain our health and vitality. Two conditions that threaten this goal are osteoporosis and heart disease, with heart disease being the number one killer of women. It makes sense, therefore, to focus on ways to prevent these conditions.

Osteoporosis

Osteoporosis, a condition characterized by low bone mass that leads to bone fragility and an increased rate of fractures, is a leading cause of suffering and disability in women. In the United States, there are at least 250,000 hip fractures each year, the majority of them in women. These fractures represent only a small proportion of the fractures caused by osteoporosis. For a 50-year-old white woman, the lifetime risk for some fractures is almost 40 percent. The rate for African American women is about a third of that, probably due to higher peak bone mass. Bone mass increases rapidly in young women, reaching a peak in their 20s and 30s. After age 35 to 40, bone mass begins to decline in both men and women, but in women, the rate of bone loss accelerates dramatically after menopause.

The number of women with osteopenia, or low bone mass (less severe than osteoporosis), may be even higher than anyone suspected. In the National Osteoporosis Risk Assessment Study, over 200,000 women over the age of 50 without known osteoporosis had bone densitometry testing. Overall, 39.6 percent were found to have low bone mass (osteopenia) and 7.2 percent had severely low bone mass, or osteoporosis. Thus, almost half of the women had unsuspected low bone mass. Both conditions lead to an increase risk of fractures in subsequent years. So clearly we want to take steps to prevent this condition.

A Lifestyle for Bone Health

When we met Christina, she was a tall, fair, 53-year-old studying oceanography. We could easily visualize her doing her favorite activity, hiking. Hiking is an ideal bone health sport because it involves weight-bearing exercise with the legs and the gear provides an upper body workout. So Christina was okay when it came to exercise. We need to remind some women who engage in spinning, biking, and running that they also need weight-bearing exercises for their arms. Such exercises include lifting free weights, doing push-ups or pull-ups, or participating in racquet sports.

Most women take in entirely too little calcium. Christina's nutritional intake was typical. Fortunately, she was only a little bit preoccupied with her weight and had not gone on any fad diets, popular with so many women and usually calcium-depriving. Still, she had eliminated dairy products because she didn't like them much. She had a vitamin-rich diet with lots of fruits and vegetables; she ate chicken and beans and "pigged out periodically with a Big Mac." A quick calculation revealed that Christina took in only about 600 milligrams of calcium a day, much less than the recommended 1,200 to 1,500 milligrams for her age. Bad news for her bones. She had a bottle of calcium tablets at home (distributed at a health fair) but usually forgot to take them. So we suggested she throw some Tums, Rolaids, or chewy chocolate candy (now you're talking!) calcium supplements into her backpack. These contain, depending upon the type and strength, 250 to 500 milligrams each (check the label for elemental calcium). No more than half of your daily requirement should be taken at one time or it won't be absorbed. The necessary 400 IU of vitamin D was easy for Christina, since it is manufactured in the skin by absorbing sunlight. Normally ten to fifteen minutes of exposure to sunlight is enough. But sunscreen, which we want you to use, interferes with this process. So most multivitamins and some calcium supplements also contain the needed 400 to 800 IUs of vitamin D.

Vitamin D helps calcium absorption. If you take calcium, but it isn't absorbed, you are not accomplishing anything. The National Osteoporosis Foundation (www.nof.org/prevention/calcium.html) puts it this way: "Vitamin D is a key that unlocks the door to allow calcium to leave the intestine and enter the bloodstream."

So Christina needed to work on her calcium intake. It can be convenient and economical to increase calcium intake by adding powdered nonfat dry milk to foods such as soups, homemade baked goods, cereals, or casseroles. One tablespoon has 52 milligrams of calcium.

Many women, sobered by their exposure to older relatives and friends who have suffered the effects of osteoporosis, have the opposite problem: They take the supplements but neglect the exercise. This may be due in part to the relative lack of school athletic programs for girls who grew up before the 1970s. Enacted in 1972, Title IX, now under attack, mandated equal opportunities and exposed girls to a whole range of team sports that earlier generations had no experience of. Still, it's never too late to start. Weight-bearing activities will pay off in the prevention of osteoporosis. Remember, you need to involve both your arms and legs. So if you're a walker, add some free weights some of the time. (Okay, so we do nag a bit.) And if you love to swim, that's fantastic for many reasons, but it's not the ideal exercise for the prevention of osteoporosis. Even though the use of your muscles in swimming does build strength, the water actually supports your weight and thus you don't get the full benefit.

Treatment

Patricia is 65, and we're amazed her osteoporosis isn't worse. She tells us how she has lost some height, but thus far has had no fractures. ("My strong Polish bones," she says, having immigrated to the United States over forty years ago.) Patricia was prescribed prednisone for asthma and has taken it on and off for thirty years. This put her at risk for osteoporosis. She also took Synthroid, having been treated successfully for thyroid cancer many years earlier. Too much Synthroid is also associated with osteoporosis, but Patricia's dose was closely monitored over the years.

In a way, Patricia is correct about her bones. She has a rosy complexion and piercing blue eyes, and is not thin. Since she is somewhat overweight and loves dairy products, she may well have had strong bones at one time. Numerous studies have shown that a higher body mass index (BMI) is protective against osteoporosis, while low body weight is a risk factor (at last some good news for larger women). Patricia also took hormone therapy for five years after menopause to treat hot flashes.

Still, the prednisone has taken its toll and she has osteoporosis. So she wanted to review her choices for treatment of osteoporosis. In the Women's Health Initiative trial, estrogen has been shown to reduce the rates of hip fractures by 34 percent and of all fractures by 24 percent. Despite these impressive results, aware of the risks of long-term HT, many experts now recommend other choices including the bisphosphonates alendronate (Fosamax), risedronate (Actonel), calcitonin, and raloxifene (Evista).

SERMs

The class of selective estrogen receptor modulators (SERMs) shows promise in the prevention of conditions associated with menopause. SERMs are medications that act *like* estrogen on some tissues and organs, but have actions *opposite* to estrogen—anti-estrogen—on others. The perfect SERM would have the good qualities of estrogen without any of the bad qualities. However, at this point the perfect SERM has not been developed. Tamoxifen and raloxifene are the two SERMs in wide use at this time. Since tamoxifen is used only for the prevention of breast cancer, we will examine it in Chapter 8.

Raloxifene

Raloxifene, or Evista, is approved for the prevention and treatment of osteoporosis. The major effects of raloxifene have been demonstrated in the MORE (Multiple Outcomes Raloxifene Effects) trial. This was a trial of nearly 8,000 postmenopausal women with osteoporosis, followed for three years on either raloxifene or placebo. The participants on raloxifene had increased bone mineral density, a 76 percent reduction in breast cancer, and improvements in their cholesterol. However, the raloxifene-treated women also had increased blood clots and hot flashes. There was no effect on the uterus. Additionally, there was no difference in cardiovascular events, as had been seen in HT. The RUTH (Raloxifene Use in the Heart) Trial is now ongoing to determine the effect of raloxifene on cardiac events in women who already have heart disease.

Raloxifene may be an option for postmenopausal women to prevent and treat osteoporosis, particularly for those women who also want to lower their risk of breast cancer. Studies have shown that raloxifene decreases spinal fractures by 30 to 50 percent. As yet, studies have not shown a decrease in hip or other fractures except those of the spine.

Bisphosphonates and Calcitonin

The bisphosphonates are approved for the prevention and treatment of osteoporosis and calcitonin is approved for treatment only. Studies have shown that the bisphosphonates alendronate (Fosamax) and risedronate (Actonel) can reduce fractures by half in both women who have had fractures in the past and those who haven't. Either medication should be taken on an empty stomach with eight ounces of water, and it is crucial to remain upright and delay eating for thirty minutes afterward. The drugs can cause an inflammation of the esophagus. Actonel is given daily and Fosamax can be used daily or once a week.

Calcitonin is a different type of medication. It reduces fractures in women with prior fractures by 35 percent. It can be taken as a nasal spray or an injection. It is usually prescribed when other medication cannot be tolerated or as an supplemental treatment.

Patricia tried raloxifene, but wasn't too thrilled about the new hot flashes. Overall, the effectiveness of the bisphosphonates seemed to her to make them a better deal than calcitonin. She agreed to take alendronate (Fosamax), 70 milligrams once a week (this dose is for osteoporosis; 35 milligrams would be required for women with osteopenia). When she learned about the potential inflammation of her esophagus, she said she'd be careful to follow all of the directions exactly: "I want to keep enjoying my food." We hoped that the medication would increase bone density and help Patricia stay healthy.

So you see, Patricia was able to think through her options and make a choice that met her needs. But what should the average woman do about osteoporosis or osteopenia? If she doesn't have low bone mass, she should be sure to get enough calcium (1,200 to 1,500 milligrams per day) with vitamin D (400 to 800 IU per day) and do those weight-bearing activities. If a woman has had any fractures or is over 65, the guidelines issued by the U.S. Preventive Services Task Force recommend a bone density test, a very low dose X-ray that measures the bone mineral density (BMD) at the spine and the hip. It is painless and accurate. The most common and well studied is the dual energy X-ray absorptiometry (DEXA). The task force does not suggest routine screening for women under age 65 unless they have had fractures or have other risk factors (in addition to menopause) for osteoporosis. Patricia should have her bone density monitored now that she has started taking medication for prevention. It is recommended that bone density be tested every two years.

And Keep Your Eye on Teriparatide

A newly approved medication, teriparatide (Forteo), is a synthetic form of parathyroid hormone, which is produced in the body and stimulates the formulation of new bone. This is the only bone-*building* drug approved to treat osteoporosis. The bisphosphonates, SERMS, and calcitonin do not build new bone but decrease the breakdown of bone. In a trial of teriparatide, it was found to be more effective than a placebo in increasing bone density and decreasing new fractures. Unlike alendronate, which can be taken as a pill, teriparatide must be taken as a daily injection. There has been concern, based on animal studies, that this medication might increase the chances of bone cancer; no cases have yet been reported from human trials.

Preventing Heart Disease: A Heart-Smart Lifestyle

At one time, heart disease was thought to be a man's problem. Now we know that although men have heart attacks at a younger age, one out of two women will die of heart disease or a stroke.

Heart disease, or cardiovascular disease, is really an umbrella term for a number of conditions involving the heart and blood vessels both inside and around the heart. The heart is basically a muscle that depends on a supply of blood delivered by blood vessels known as coronary arteries. If these vessels become narrowed, they may not carry an adequate supply of blood for the heart muscle to function optimally. When blood flow is limited, it can result in a reversible injury known as ischemia. Chest pain, or angina, is the usual symptom of ischemia. Ischemia can progress to an irreversible injury known as myocardial infarction, or heart attack. Chest pain that persists may indicate irreversible damage and should always be evaluated. If enough of the heart muscle is affected, the heart may not pump properly and fluid can accumulate in the lungs, resulting in congestive heart failure.

Some risk factors for heart disease are beyond our control: for example, being African American or having a family history of heart disease (in a father, brother, uncle, or grandfather before the age of 55 or a mother, sister, aunt, or grandmother before the age of 65). But there's a lot we can do to influence other important risk factors: smoking; having a sedentary lifestyle, diabetes, high blood pressure, or elevated cholesterol; being overweight; and experiencing high levels of stress.

We understand how difficult it is to change behaviors. Dieting, increasing one's exercise, and quitting smoking are not easy. Our goal in this chapter is *not* to make you feel guilty. Rather, we want to demystify the process of change to make it seem less overwhelming.

We don't just wake up one morning and change. Rather, change is a process and involves a series of stages. A team of psychologists led by James O. Prochaska, Ph.D., developed the Stages of Change Model. The model has revolutionized the treatment of addictive behaviors by helping us understand how people change. The stages are precontemplation, contemplation, preparation, action, and maintenance. Precontemplation is the stage when a person denies that she has a problem or may be unaware of the negative consequences of her behavior. A woman in this stage may also be demoralized and have given up hope. Therefore people in this stage do not intend to change during the foreseeable future. People in the contemplation stage may recognize the need to change. However, they may be ambivalent and are not ready to take action immediately. Those in the preparation stage intend to change during the next month and have begun to take small steps toward their goals. The action stage involves modifying problematic behaviors and/or developing new, healthier behaviors. Finally, the maintenance stage involves sustaining the changes for at least six months.

An important part of the Stages of Change Model is the understanding that the change process is a spiral. Change is not linear, but may involve several relapses before it becomes permanent. So if you are attempting to change, know that it may take time, but by using the model and learning from it you will be able to succeed in the long run.

The Stages of Change Model can be applied to smoking, the number one preventable risk for heart disease. A smoker who says "Smoking is fine" or gives examples of nonsmokers who have had heart attacks is in the precontemplation stage. This person has little awareness of her danger and she has no intention of quitting smoking. She needs help in understanding the risks of smoking as well as the process of not smoking.

Contemplation occurs when a person is aware of the problem but has not yet planned to quit. She is beginning to think about quitting. "Smoking is causing me some breathing problems. Maybe I should quit."

The planning stage may well be the most important one and involves setting a quit date for smoking, telling friends and family, and eliminating any cues associated with smoking. The woman may need to find another tool to manage stress.

Maintaining change is key and also takes work and determination. A person can relapse at any point in the process, but even though she may backslide, she probably won't go all the way back to the precontemplation stage. Difficult life changes may require multiple attempts before the change becomes permanent. With smoking, for example, the chance that someone will successfully quit becomes better with each attempt. Practice really does make perfect.

This model has been beneficial to many of our patients thinking about preventing heart disease. It combines a scientific "what works" approach with the patience required to make lasting changes. You might want to read the details in *Changing for Good*, the excellent book by Dr. Prochaska, John Norcross, Ph.D., and Carlo DiClemente, Ph.D. It is wise to tackle one behavior at a time rather than attempting a major overhaul all at once. The changes to make follow.

Stop Smoking

If you smoke, you probably know that in addition to damaging your cardiovascular system, you run the risk of developing emphysema and several types of cancer—including lung cancer, cancers of the head and neck, and bladder cancer. Your secondhand smoke may also harm people around you. You probably believe that you can't stop. You can. It is incredibly difficult, but you can quit. Maybe this fact will motivate you: Your risk of developing heart disease will drop to where it would have been if you'd never smoked within one to five years after you've quit.

In choosing a smoking cessation program, remember that women have different reasons for smoking. Many women use smoking to control their appetites, to cope with stress, or even to treat depressive symptoms. Look for a smoking cessation program that addresses the specific reasons you smoke. For example, many programs recommend increased exercise or relaxation training. Both the American Cancer Society (www.cancer.org) and the American Heart Association (www.americanheart.org) offer excellent programs. The Center for Disease Control also offers the "You Can Quit Smoking Guide." University- or medical-school-affiliated clinics often offer research programs that may be free or for a minimal charge.

Study after study has shown that there are several key ingredients for success in quitting smoking. These include being motivated to quit, setting a quit date, restructuring your environment, using nicotine replacement or a medication to deal with the physical addiction in some cases, and planning for difficult situations.

Motivating yourself involves the many good reasons that you want to quit smoking. These could include, in addition to the health benefits we've listed, the health of your loved ones, the extra money you'll save, and your appearance (fewer wrinkles, unstained hands and teeth).

Once you've set a quit date, it's time to change your environment. Recent research suggests that the elimination of cigarettes from your environment is the most powerful component of the plan. Get rid of every last cigarette and ashtray in your home, workplace, and car. Check those jacket pockets and hiding places, too. Ask others not to smoke in your home. Most people prefer to quit smoking cold turkey—completely at once. To make it easier, though, you might start to cut down gradually before your actual quit date. There is no single right way. Try to apply what you've learned from all those past attempts so that this will be the last time you have to go through this.

Most people stop the *act* of smoking, but many need nicotine replacement in order to avoid the physical withdrawal. Nicotine is as addictive as cocaine or heroin. In addition, if you are a regular smoker, nicotine or its by-products can remain in your body for three or four days. The good news is that although withdrawal symptoms can last for several weeks, they are usually at their worst at 48 to 72 hours. Nicotine replacement now comes in many forms, including patches, gum, nasal sprays, and lozenges. Your physician may also prescribe an antidepressant medication, bupropion or Zyban (also marketed for depression as Wellbutrin). Even before it has a chance to act as an antidepressant, this helps to decrease cigarette craving. In one study, 36 percent of people using the nicotine patch and 49 percent of people taking bupropion were able to quit smoking for a month. When the two methods were combined, the rate jumped to 50 percent.

When times are tough, the American Cancer Society recommends the Four As: avoidance, altering your environment, alternatives, and activities. So you might need more exercise to burn off steam or chewing gum to deal with your habit. Some people like to rub a smooth stone or squeeze a stress ball (springy rubber ball) to keep their hands occupied. You can do it. Remember, the goal is to stay off cigarettes. Mark Twain said, "Quitting smoking is easy. I've done it a thousand times." Keep trying; it's worth it.

Get Some Exercise

You probably have heard and read a lot about this, so we'll just review some basic principles.

- Get moving. For optimum heart protection, 30 to 60 minutes of moderately aerobic exercise on most days of the week is recommended. Your exercise is moderately aerobic if you sweat, are breathless, or feel fatigued. One rule of thumb is that if you are talking a lot while walking, you are not walking fast enough! Examples include dancing, brisk walking (3 to 4 miles per hour), and even active yard work.
- You can break up periods of exercise into smaller amounts of time.
- Something is better than nothing. Check with your health care professional to help you assess your level of fitness and the appropriateness of any plan.
- Try to have fun. If you take the time to find an activity you enjoy, you'll be more likely to stick with it.
- Okay, let's say that it is *not* that much fun. Then pair your exercise with something that is pleasurable. If you have a friend who is in the same boat (and who isn't?), try out different classes together—spinning, yoga, or Pilates are some possibilities—and then chose your favorite to continue. If you prefer solo activities, add some headphones or read while you're on the treadmill.
- If you can afford it, schedule a few sessions with a personal trainer. You can learn about proper technique and different types of exercise that will help you stay motivated. This doesn't have to cost a fortune. Many gyms, Ys, and community centers employ trainers. Schedule a few sessions and then periodic boosters. Besides keeping you motivated, such sessions are useful in monitoring your progress.

- Variety, or cross-training, can help maintain your interest as well as improve your overall fitness. So mix it up. Don't do the same activity every day. Do weight training Monday, Wednesday, and Friday, and take brisk walks on Tuesday, Thursday, and Saturday. (And on the seventh day, she rested.)
- If you've decided to exercise, let's say, five to six days a week, try to make a plan and stick to it. Don't wait until the alarm clock awakens you to decide that you'll jog this morning. It's much harder to make a new decision every day than to do it just once. Have your gear ready the night before so you are ready to go.
- Physical activity, not just organized sports or exercise, is also important. You may have seen people wearing small pedometers on their shoes, arms, belts, or waistbands. They are trying to increase the distance they walk or the number of steps they take in a day. Let's say one day you walk 2,000 steps, or about a mile. Try to increase it. Take the stairs, not the elevator. Find the parking spot farthest away. Mall-walk. Choose walking over driving. The pedometer, by giving you immediate feedback, can make it fun and challenging.

You'll read more in Chapter 7 about Cheryl, a woman who increased her exercise level. But until then, here is just a partial list of health benefits of regular exercise, in addition to preventing cardiovascular disease: prevention of osteoporosis, weight loss, reduction in body fat, blood pressure control, an improved cholesterol profile, improved mood, better quality of life, longer life. You get the idea? Go for it.

Treat Medical Conditions

Hypertension, or High Blood Pressure Hypertension, or high blood pressure, is defined as blood pressure greater than 140/90 mm Hg. The first number, 140, is your systolic pressure, or the maximum pressure when the heart beats. Diastolic blood pressure, or 90 in this case, means the minimum blood pressure when the heart is in between beats. Optimal blood pressure is less than 120/80 mm Hg. Blood pressure is considered high normal when it is 130–139/85–89 mm Hg. A new classification of blood pressure has been introduced. It is called "prehypertension" and includes blood pressure of 120–139/80–89 mm Hg. People with a family history of high blood pressure, African American women, and women over the age of 55 are more likely to develop hypertension.

Exercise, weight loss, salt restriction, and alcohol restriction can all help lower blood pressure, as can several types of blood pressure medications. The most commonly used medications include water pills, or diuretics, ACE (angiotensin-converting enzyme) inhibitors, calcium channel blockers, and beta-blockers. You and your physician need to find the best treatment for you, depending on any other medical conditions that you might have, the side effects of the various types of medications, and their effect on your blood pressure.

Remember that hypertension is a silent killer—that is, it can have no symptoms. So have your blood pressure checked regularly.

Cholesterol More than a third of American women are at increased risk of heart attacks because of high cholesterol levels. Cholesterol circulates in the bloodstream and is found in certain foods. Simply put, there are two major components of cholesterol to consider. The first type is LDL, or low-density lipoprotein, which is referred to as the "bad" cholesterol. The second type is HDL, or high-density lipoprotein, or "good" cholesterol. High levels of overall cholesterol, especially LDL, are associated with the buildup of fatty deposits in the arteries. Hardening of the arteries, called atherosclerosis, occurs when blood flow slows down due to these clogged arteries.

To reduce cholesterol levels, you should change to a low-fat, low-cholesterol diet; lose or control your weight; and increase exercise. There are also medications to reduce cholesterol. These are referred to as the statins and are highly effective in reducing cholesterol in many people. Your response to any of these measures will depend largely on the type of cholesterol problem that you have. Don't be discouraged if the "perfect" diet doesn't lower your cholesterol enough. It is not a sign of failure on your part. Some people simply need medication to get their cholesterol in the right range.

Triglycerides Triglycerides are another type of fat in the blood. A normal range of triglycerides is 85 to 250 mg/dL. High levels of triglycerides may be associated with other conditions such as diabetes or they may be an inherited problem. Diet, weight loss, and limiting alcohol can help reduce triglycerides. There are also medications that can specifically lower triglycerides if they remain high.

Diabetes Diabetes mellitus puts a woman at increased risk for heart disease. Diabetes occurs when the body does not make enough insulin or does not use insulin effectively. Insulin is a hormone that processes and stores sugar. When insulin doesn't work, sugar levels in the blood become elevated. The best test to detect diabetes is a blood test. A fasting blood sugar (taken twelve hours after the last meal or beverage) level of 126 or more mg/dL indicates diabetes. Sometimes a glucose tolerance test is checked to detect diabetes as well. Diabetes speeds up the process of atherosclerosis, leading to heart disease. It can also affect blood supply to the extremities, kidney function, sensation, vision, and the ability to fight infection.

If you have a family history of diabetes or symptoms including frequent urination, excessive thirst, weight loss, or persistent vaginal yeast infections, be sure to tell your doctor so you can be tested. Diabetes can be effectively treated and the health consequences minimized.

So to prevent heart disease, we need to stop smoking, treat any relevant medical condition, exercise, and let's see, what else? We've deliberately left alcohol for one of the last topics.

Alcohol

Let's face it, we'd all love a magic bullet. It would be so much easier to have a glass of wine or take a pill than to do the hard work of restricting calories, exercising more, or quitting smoking. There is some evidence that people who drink alcohol in moderation have a lower risk of heart disease than those who don't drink at all or those who drink excessively. The problem, however, is that this evidence is drawn nearly exclusively from observational studies, which means that these free-range people chose to drink or not. Like the hormone-heart connection, it is possible that drinking alcohol in moderation may be associated with other behaviors that really are heart healthy, such as exercise or low-fat diets. To conclude that people who don't drink should start drinking is a real leap from these studies, and it may well be a dangerous one. What about drinking and driving? What about liver disease?

There may be some serious health consequences to what most

people consider moderate drinking, especially for women, who are more susceptible to the effects of alcohol than men. In fact, more than one drink per day is potentially hazardous for women, putting them at increased risk of liver disease and breast cancer. The bottom line is that for women, it is probably okay to continue to drink if you drink one or fewer drinks per day and no more than three drinks on any occasion. If you drink more than this, you should cut down. If you don't drink now, don't start.

Dieting and Weight Loss

Now that you are warmed up, here's another fun subject. Most women know a lot about diets and calories. But recently there has been even more controversy over the best diet for heart health. Here is our strategy based on our take on the controversy. First, identify your goals. If you are in good health but want to lose weight, there is only one answer. You need to take in fewer calories than you burn. Since a pound of weight equals 3,500 calories, you'll need to take in 500 fewer calories or burn off 500 extra calories per day to lose a pound a week (7 days × 500 calories = 3,500 calories). As to what type of diet you choose, the trade-off is between losing enough weight to keep you motivated and being able to stay on the plan.

There is great debate about the merits of the high-protein diets (Atkins); the typical more balanced lower-calorie, low-fat diet; and the very low fat diets (Ornish). Dr. Dean Ornish's low-fat diet has been helpful to people with a diagnosis of heart disease. Dr. Atkins's diet has helped people who haven't been able to lose enough weight quickly. However, if you have been advised to watch your cholesterol and your consumption of fat, you should check in with your health professional before starting this diet. While many people can lose a lot of weight on the Atkins diet, they have trouble maintaining the total lack of carbohydrates.

Here are a few other considerations. If your goal is not only to lose weight but also to improve your heart health, you really do need to watch the fat. Dr. Walter Willett, the senior researcher of the Nurses' Health Study, recommends a change from the U.S. Department of Agriculture's Food Pyramid (www.health.gov/dietaryguidelines). Dr.

Willett's book *Eat, Drink, and Be Healthy: The Harvard Medical School Guide to Healthy Eating*, published in 2001, modifies the traditional food pyramid, separating out red meat from other proteins and bad fats from good fats. The Healthy Eating Pyramid also recommends whole grain rather than refined carbohydrates. Too many people replace all the fat they cut out with refined carbohydrates and sugars. This can lead to peaks and valleys in blood sugar and the quick return of hunger.

A similar approach is taken by *Low Fat Lies, High Fat Frauds, and the Best Diet in the World* by Mary Flynn and Kevin Vigilante, M.D. They recommend the Mediterranean diet, one rich in fruits, vegetables, and whole grains. They emphasize olive oil as a good type of fat and point out that some fat helps you feel full. This helps you stay on a diet.

Finally, Dr. Barbara Rolls in *The Volumetric's Weight-Control Plan* recommends foods that have low energy density—that is, have lots of water. So soups, stews, and high-fiber foods high in water content are recommended. You can eat 2 cups of grapes, a low energy density food; but less than a ¼ cup of high-density raisins for an equivalent 100 calories. Besides, eating grapes takes longer (particularly if you peel them) and makes you feel fuller.

The best plans emphasize fruits, vegetables, and whole grains. All such plans focus on good fats versus bad fats. All such plans rely largely on common sense. The problem, of course, comes in sticking to the plan.

Midlife is an especially difficult time to lose weight. The average woman gains 8 to 10 pounds during the decade between 45 and 55. (Yes, it is sad but true.) At one time people believed estrogen therapy was the culprit, but this has been shown to be false (although estrogen can lead to water retention and breast tenderness). The culprit seems to be a change in metabolism that occurs with aging. Seems unfair, doesn't it?

You'll lose weight and feel better if you combine a reasonable nutritional program, such as those described above, with exercise. Another tip is to get social support. One reason for the success of group weight-loss programs is that being with other people with similar issues is therapeutic. This may be especially true for overweight middle-aged women, who continue to be stigmatized. Watch any television program, listen to talk radio, go to the movies, and you'll see the antifat bias is one of the last socially acceptable prejudices. Even movies like *The Nutty Professor* and *Shallow Hal*, supposedly sensitive to overweight people, use a nasty new formula: a hundred minutes of fat jokes, ten minutes of apologies. Not fair. Not cool. Not funny.

Stress Management

Relax. We hope we haven't stressed you with too many ideas about heart health. If anything, we want to help you reduce your stress because stress reduction is good for your heart, too. The relationship between stress and heart disease is complex. We are only now sorting out the psychological issues for women because most of the research conducted before the 1980s was done only on (surprise!) men.

Stress management courses teach you ways to reduce your stressful reactions as they are manifested in thoughts, beliefs, emotions, and behavior. To understand physiological stress, imagine that you are driving down a highway at night. Let's say the traffic is light and you are enjoying the ride, feeling relaxed. All of a sudden an animal darts out in front of you. Your resulting gasp and increase in muscle tension and heart rate are classic physiological stress responses.

Everyday stress can produce the same wear and tear, to a lesser degree, on your system. These are often reactions to behavior and involve your thoughts, feelings, and belief systems. For this reason, most stress management programs now include a cognitive approach as well as progressive muscle relaxation. For example, suppose you work in sales and you receive a report that indicates that your sales are down. You might have a resulting thought: "I will be fired soon." This could, in turn, set off an old negative belief: "I'm not a good employee anyway and I'm bound to be a failure."

Cognitive therapy (also called cognitive behavior therapy, or CBT) can help you analyze this chain of stress. First, your negative appraisal and general belief will be challenged. Is there evidence that you will be fired? Is this the first bad month you've had? Does anyone else have the same or similar figures? The therapist or course leader will also interpret the automatic connections that end in "I am bound to be a failure." Are there steps you can take to improve your work? Do you have other value in your company? And even in the worst-case scenario, if you did lose your job, would that make you a failure as a person?

This systematic challenging of automatic negative thoughts and beliefs is a primary part of cognitive therapy. Over time, you learn to challenge thoughts and beliefs and self-correct. This helps reduce stress and opens the door to enhanced problem-solving skills.

If you've already had a heart attack or developed risks for heart disease, stress management is particularly important. See the Resources section at the back of the book. Be sure to look for a book or program that addresses women's issues. For example, men who've had heart attacks can take time off from work. Yet a woman, employed or not, is rarely able to "take time off" from household and caregiving responsibilities. Groups of other women are better able to give support, advice, and encouragement. Sisterhood remains powerful in midlife and beyond.

And Keep Your Eye On . . .

At one time, social scientists believed that there were two personality types, Type A and Type B, that were relevant to heart disease. Type A people were aggressive and hard-driving, whereas Type Bs were calmer and less competitive. Doctors found that Type A personalities—men, actually, since the research focused only on them—were more prone to heart disease.

Over time, however, even with men, it became clear that this analysis was too simplistic. Not *all* aspects of the Type A personalities proved to be detrimental. People who experience negative emotions, especially anger, are more prone to heart disease. When the negative emotion is turned inward, it is now labeled the Type D, or distressed, personality.

In one study performed in England, the death rate from cardiovascular disease was much higher for those with Type D personalities than for others. This was extremely significant, with 27 percent of the Type Ds dying within a seven- to nine-year period, compared to 7 percent of the others. Remember from Chapter 2 that a result is considered significant when the result is reported as having a probability, or p-value, of less than .05? Well, in this study, even when they controlled the other factors, the results were significant at the level of $p<.0004$! Impressive.

Other research suggests that even anger expressed *outwardly* puts a person at risk. A study of women who tended to be angry found that when they were deliberately annoyed during an experiment (psychologists can be tricky!), their systolic blood pressure increased more than that of women who did not tend to be angry. Finally, even the wives of angry men suffered, with another study finding that women married to angry men showed large increases in blood pressure during discussions of marital stress.

What to do about anger, then? Current research is helping people identify angry feelings and learn better coping and problem-solving skills. The belief is that it is the sustained high level of arousal that accompanies the anger (blood pressure, heart rate) that may be detrimental. Therefore, learning to be flexible, to express feelings constructively, and then to let go may ultimately be found to protect the heart.

Other areas of research in women with heart disease concerns work and marital stress. The Stockholm Female Coronary Risk Study found that marital stress worsened the prognosis for women with coronary disease. Stress in a relationship, rather than work stress, was highly correlated with repeated coronary events. What's going on here? The Stockholm study also found that depressive symptoms were twice as common in women with coronary disease, compared to those without. It is quite possible that depression, or at least depressed mood, is the link. Does marital stress lead to depression, which leads to coronary disease? Or does depression lead to both marital stress and coronary disease? We know for sure that coronary disease can lead to depression. Whatever the specific cause, we know that treatment for depression does help.

C-Reactive Protein (CRP) Screening

Here's a problem. One quarter of the people who have heart attacks have no known risk factors. New research suggests that inflammation may be a better predictor than elevated cholesterol of cardiovascular problems in women. C-reactive protein (CRP) reflects inflammation in the body. Normally, inflammation is part of a healthy process that triggers the immune system to help the body heal. But if something goes wrong, inflammation can injure tissue. In addition, inflammation can negatively affect the fatty buildup or plaque that clogs arteries.

One study followed 28,000 women for eight years; half of the 28,000 had experienced heart attacks and/or strokes and had low levels of LDL cholesterol. In contrast, women who had high levels of CRP were more likely to have heart attacks. The American Heart Association and the Centers for Disease Control have agreed that people already at some risk for heart disease may benefit from CRP screening. A randomized controlled study will compare rosuvastatin, one of the medications that lowers cholesterol, with a placebo in the prevention of heart disease. The subjects will have low LDL levels (below 130 mg/dL) and high CRP values (above 2 mg/dL). The researchers will examine the effect on heart disease. So stay tuned to see if CRP screening is added to cholesterol for routine screening.

○─○─○

CHAPTER FIVE

Not Your Average
Menopause:

Surgical Menopause and Breast Cancer Survivors

Natural menopause is a gradual process that does not neces-sarily provoke a medical or psychological crisis. Each individual woman has a unique menopausal transition based on her medical and psychological history, resources available, and to a certain extent, chance. For example, if you are an active executive with good health insurance and a few hot flashes, you may have one type of menopause. If, on the other hand, you are a recently divorced, unemployed woman with a history of depression, the challenges of menopause and midlife may be much greater.

In addition, several medical conditions affect menopause. These include thyroid disease and premature ovarian failure (when menopause occurs before the age of 40). Chemotherapy and/or radiation treatment can cause menopause. More dramatically, surgical removal of the ovaries leads to immediate menopause, as can the treatment of breast cancer.

Hysterectomy refers to the surgical removal of the uterus and cervix. Oophorectomy is the surgical removal of the ovaries. By the age of 60, one out of four American women has had a hysterectomy. It is the second most common surgery performed on women (cesarean section is the most common), and 600,000 hysterectomies are performed annually in the United States. The United States has one of the highest rates of hysterectomy in the world: 5 in 1,000 women annually. In England, the rate is less than 3 per 1,000 women annually, and in Norway, less than 2 in 1,000. There are also regional differences within the United States, with the South having the highest rate. A hysterectomy may be done with an abdominal incision (abdominal hysterectomy) or a vaginal incision (vaginal hysterectomy). A laparoscopic hysterectomy is surgery using a flexible instrument inserted through a small abdominal incision.

Of the women having hysterectomies, 55 percent also have their ovaries removed. If a premenopausal woman has an oophorectomy, she goes through menopause immediately because the ovaries, the primary organs producing estrogen, are gone. Women who have had a hysterectomy but *not* an oophorectomy still go through a natural menopause. However, since the uterus has been removed, they have no menstrual cycles. Therefore, since there are no periods to become irregular, it is more difficult to identify perimenopause.

Hysterectomies and oophorectomies are somewhat controversial within the field of medicine. There is no doubt that for some time they were done unnecessarily and that alternative treatments were not explored. On the other hand, Drs. Carlson, Nichols, and Schiff, authors of one of the landmark studies of hysterectomy, published in 1993, found that most women felt significant improvement afterward because their symptoms were alleviated. This finding has been confirmed in more recent studies as well.

Over 50 percent of hysterectomies are performed because of endometriosis or fibroids. Endometriosis is a condition in which the lining of the uterus is found in other abdominal organs. Fibroids, or leiomyomas, are noncancerous growths in the tissue of the wall of the uterus. Both of these conditions can be uncomfortable and painful. Other conditions that lead to elective hysterectomy are dysfunctional uterine bleeding, endometrial hyperplasia, and chronic pelvic pain.

There are now numerous alternatives to hysterectomy. For example, fibroids can be removed surgically without removing the uterus. This procedure is called a myomectomy. Dysfunctional uterine bleeding, endometriosis, and endometrial hyperplasia can respond to hormonal treatments and new procedures. And even if a hysterectomy is selected as the optimal treatment, an oophorectomy is not always necessary.

In the past physicians might have found it easier to recommend oophorectomies because it was assumed that all women would take estrogen therapy afterward. Given the recent concerns about estrogen, however, there might be cause to reconsider. This will depend on the results of that part of the Women's Health Initiative studying women on estrogen alone, scheduled to be completed in 2005.

Chronic pelvic pain can sometimes lead to hysterectomy. This is a very complicated condition that requires *both* a psychological and a medical evaluation. All too often a woman has either one or the other. The need for a psychological assessment is clear: Pain that influences sexuality requires an exploration of an individual's family and social history, attitudes, and values. Sexual or physical abuse can lead to pelvic pain.

On the other hand, women who have histories of psychological or physical abuse also suffer from medical problems. So a woman should not accept an "it must be stress" approach unless she has had a thorough gynecological evaluation. Women with endometriosis, for example, have often been stigmatized as having psychologically based pain before an accurate diagnosis was made. So a comprehensive assessment is optimal. Like other forms of chronic pain, chronic pelvic pain is often best treated using a multidisciplinary approach.

A hysterectomy is sometimes necessary, especially in a medical emergency such as a massive hemorrhage, a ruptured uterus, uncontrollable infection, or invasive uterine cancer.

All too often women who are about to have a hysterectomy are told, "Let's get rid of your ovaries, too. You don't need them anymore anyway." This may be true if a woman is a certain age and has completed her family, but remember, there are other positive effects of estrogen. Dr. Carlson and associates suggest that "oophorectomy is recommended for women over 50 when a hysterectomy is performed, whereas the ovaries should be conserved if a woman is under 45. However, they recommend that the woman's "risk of ovarian cancer and her ability to take estrogen replacement therapy" should also be considered.

With respect to oophorectomy, certainly ovarian cancer would require surgery. There are other times when a woman may choose to have her ovaries removed as a preventive measure. This would be true when a woman has the BRCA gene related to ovarian and breast cancer. Women with this gene or those with more than two first-degree relatives with ovarian cancer may face a lifetime risk of 10 to 25 percent of developing ovarian cancer.

The perimenopausal woman who does have a hysterectomy and oophorectomy is sent directly to menopause; she does not pass go. Thus she is much more likely than a woman experiencing natural menopause to have severe hot flashes. Additionally, she is now at higher risk of developing osteoporosis. Many experts agree that estrogen therapy should be instituted and continued until the age at which menopause would have occurred naturally, usually around age 51.

Rita was lucky. We met her at one of our town meetings and she told us this story. When she was 51, she noticed some spotting between her periods. She didn't call her doctor because her periods had become irregular a year earlier and she figured it was part of perimenopause. (Bad idea. Bleeding *between* actual periods means that you should call your doctor to rule out uterine cancer.) A couple of months later, Rita doubled over from pain in her pelvic area. Taken to the emergency room, she had immediate surgery that revealed fibroid uterine cancer as well as an ovarian tumor. Fortunately, the ovarian growth, although cancerous, was contained. It had twisted, cutting off her blood supply and causing the pain. Rita awakened to discover that she'd had both ovaries and her uterus removed.

Even though she was fast-forwarded to menopause, Rita realized that she'd been fortunate to dodge the bullet of ovarian cancer, which often has no symptoms. In addition to cancer treatment by her oncologist, Rita was prescribed an estrogen patch for six months because of severe hot flashes. Now, ten years later, she is cancer-free and healthy.

Depression and Oophorectomy

The surgical removal of the ovaries can be quite disruptive to a woman's life. The hormonal changes are dramatic. If the hysterectomy is performed abdominally, rather than vaginally or laparoscopically, it can require several months of recovery. In addition, some women, especially younger women, feel a sense of loss. This may be the actual loss of the ability to bear a child or the symbolic loss of her femininity. If a woman does not have the support of her family and friends, she can become isolated and withdrawn.

Yet hysterectomy and oophorectomy do not necessarily lead to depression. The results of two studies are helpful in understanding the relationship. Dr. Carlson and her colleagues did not find that women who had this surgery automatically became depressed. In contrast, many of them were relieved because the symptoms that led to the surgery were gone. However, an article by John and Sonja McKinlay and Nancy Avis of the Massachusetts Women's Health Study showed that although natural menopause was not associated with depression, surgical menopause was. Approximately 18 percent of the women who had a hysterectomy and oophorectomy were depressed. The McKinlay group studied women over a long period of time, between the ages of 45 and 55. Therefore they were able to examine the situations of the depressed women. Closer examination revealed that many of the women were depressed both before and after the surgery. It is likely that for a depressed woman, surgical menopause would exacerbate the mood problems.

Another possible explanation for the rate of depression in this study might be the underlying condition that led to the hysterectomy and oophorectomy. It is possible that in some cases the women's depression led them to experience more gynecological pain or to have an increased sensitivity to symptoms, making them more likely to have surgery than women who were not depressed. In addition, chronic pelvic pain has been associated with both depression and a history of sexual abuse. Moreover, removal of the ovaries eliminates not only the body's source of estrogen but also the major source of testosterone, which can lead to a decrease in libido. So in this situation, surgery could be unnecessary and harmful.

If you are considering surgical removal of the ovaries and uterus, we recommend the following:

- First, get a second opinion. Surgery is a significant medical decision usually requiring anesthesia and hospitalization. Ask whether there are nonsurgical treatments available for the condition. Endometriosis can be treated with a hormonal medication, just to name one example.

- Choose a surgeon who has performed many hysterectomies and oophorectomies. You want a surgeon who specializes in this area.
- Talk to a woman who has had the same surgery. She can fill you in on the details—how it feels, what to expect, how long recovery will take, and so forth.
- Estrogen therapy may well be helpful, especially on a short-term basis. Again, the hot flashes associated with surgical menopause can be more severe and frequent than those associated with natural menopause. If you find yourself sad, negative, and weepy for more than two weeks, consider an evaluation for depression. Early identification and treatment can help you feel better quickly.
- Take it easy during recovery. Although you want to get some physical activity as soon as possible, don't overdo it. Too many women resume their responsibilities as soon as they can get up. You deserve to be treated with the same care and support that you would give to others. Take it slow and allow yourself time to recover.

Breast Cancer Survivors

Diane has been coming to see us on and off for years. She now looks back on her perimenopausal years as a living hell. Diane was a talented and successful commercial artist. She'd been married to a moody and impulsive man, Geoffrey, for many years. Although Diane had been in psychotherapy, Geoffrey flatly refused counseling of any kind. They had a daughter, Genevieve, whom Diane tried to protect from her husband's irritable outbursts, with a fair degree of success. She and Genevieve shared many interests and Genevieve was a good student and musician.

When Diane began to have severe hot flashes and her periods became irregular, at age 46, she knew she was in the perimenopausal phase. As it is for many women, this phase was an existential wake-up call. Diane felt that she was entering midlife, a new stage in her life. She worried that her time for happiness was running out. After some time, she informed Geoffrey that she wanted a divorce but wanted to share custody of Genevieve. Geoffrey was furious and seemed shocked. Yet within a few weeks of the separation, he had begun dating.

The divorce process was now under way. Then in the midst of the turmoil, Diane found a lump. She had stage 1 breast cancer (localized, less than 2 centimeters in diameter large). After exploring her options, she felt the combination of lumpectomy, chemotherapy, and radiation seemed to be the most reasonable choice.

"Six weeks into chemo and I felt like a crazy person." Diane has a flair for the dramatic, but her description reveals her plight. The chemotherapy had fast-forwarded her into menopause and her hot flashes were unbearable. Since Diane's tumor was estrogen receptor positive, she would need to take tamoxifen for the next five years, which also could worsen her hot flashes. Most nights, her hot flashes were so severe that she got only a few hours of sleep. She also felt out of control, upset, and tearful. "I'd chosen to lose my husband, but I didn't expect to be sick and to feel so, well, unhinged."

Fortunately, Diane had a tremendous amount of support. She was close to several other families in the neighborhood; they could help out with the house and Genevieve could spend some nights with friends. Diane also trusted her oncologist, who was available and supportive. To control her hot flashes and treat any depressive symptoms, Diane took venlafaxine (Effexor). After six weeks, some hot flashes remained, but they were less frequent and Diane felt much better.

Now, seven years later, Diane looks back and wonders how she got through it all. In her life, the breast cancer had been the proverbial straw that broke the camel's back. The divorce was a major change, but Diane had unconsciously been moving in that direction for years. Really, she and Genevieve had led a life parallel to Geoffrey's. He moved away within a year of the divorce ("Met a younger woman— why am I not surprised?"). Diane suggested that Genevieve get some counseling, since she did miss her father, and Genevieve benefited tremendously from good, solid relationships with a few male teachers and music instructors

Meanwhile, Diane went back to school part-time, ultimately got an MBA, and now is a vice president in a large corporation. Genevieve is off at college and sees both of her parents. She has expressed some doubts about finding a reliable man and getting married and is still in psychotherapy.

Moral of the story? Diane says, "Don't get a divorce and breast cancer in the same year!" Good advice, but just as she could not predict her cancer, most women cannot plan their lives perfectly. Induced menopause may cause more severe symptoms than natural menopause does, but that doesn't mean you are crazy. As you would in the case of any serious illness, focus on rest and recovery and let your friends and family help out.

If you've had breast cancer or an oophorectomy, the suddenness of menopause may well precipitate numerous psychological and social adjustments or crises. If you are also coping with cancer, there is undoubtedly also a fear of death and suffering. Some women turn to their religious or spiritual communities for consolation and support. Support groups are also extremely helpful; sometimes just sharing your story with a woman who's been there can provide a healthy connection. Check out the Resources at the end of this book.

Breast Cancer Treatment and Menopause

Women who are undergoing treatment for breast cancer are confronted by a sometimes confusing and overwhelming array of decisions, specialists, and procedures. Therefore, it is even more important to have a physician who can organize, direct, and communicate.

Breast cancer is diagnosed in approximately 250,000 women in the United States every year. The good news is that most of these women, like Diane, will be cured. On the way to the cure, however, women must face many medical and psychological challenges. Women who were diagnosed with breast cancer before they are menopausal will have different experiences from those who were diagnosed after menopause.

Not all breast cancers are alike. Some are estrogen receptor positive tumors, which means that any additional estrogen could stimulate the cancer to spread. Even for estrogen receptor negative tumors, it is advisable to avoid hormones. This will affect the options that breast cancer survivors have for treating menopausal symptoms.

Chemotherapy, which is often used to treat breast cancer, frequently causes menopause for women over the age of 40. For women younger than 40, periods may stop temporarily. These women are also likely to have an earlier menopause. In addition to a woman's age, the dose and type of chemotherapy will determine the effect on hormonal status and onset of menopause.

All of these elements contribute to women with breast cancer experiencing more severe symptoms of menopause. The toxic effects of chemotherapy on the ovaries result in a sudden drop in estrogen levels. Thus, these women are much more like women who have had a surgical menopause than like those who have had a natural, more gradual decline in estrogen.

Use of the medication tamoxifen involves some very good news, but a little bad news. You may recall from Chapter 3 that the first SERM to be developed was tamoxifen. Tamoxifen's major benefit is its anti-estrogenic effect on breast tissue, which has led to its use in the prevention of breast cancer. Tamoxifen has been shown to reduce the risk of *first* breast cancers in women who are high risk. It also reduces the risk of second breast cancers in breast cancer patients by approximately half. Additionally, it has been shown to act like estrogen on cholesterol, by increasing the good cholesterol and decreasing the bad. Tamoxifen's effect on bone is similar to but less than that of estrogen. However, it is not FDA-approved for the prevention or treatment of osteoporosis. Still, it is a good idea to have periodic monitoring with bone density testing.

The bad news is that tamoxifen also acts as an anti-estrogen, worsening and increasing the frequency of hot flashes. This is true even in women well past menopause. The hope is that hot flashes become less pronounced after several months of tamoxifen therapy. For women experiencing tamoxifen-induced hot flashes, there may be a light at the end of the tunnel because treatment with tamoxifen usually lasts for no more than five years. Because there is an increased risk of uterine cancer with tamoxifen, any vaginal bleeding should be reported immediately. Yearly gynecological exams are also mandatory.

Given the severity of hot flashes in breast cancer survivors, it should be no surprise that most of the studies of nonhormonal treatments have been done on this highly motivated group of women. This makes it very easy to apply the study results to the specific situation of breast cancer. In general, options for treatment of hot flashes for breast cancer survivors include everything except estrogen and estrogen-like medications. As with women who want to avoid the hormonal treatment of hot flashes, a good strategy is to start with vitamin E and behavioral and lifestyle changes. This can be done before making any additional decisions. Your physician should work with you on the choices. Sometimes the choice of the prescription medication to treat hot flashes is made easier because of another health concern such as depression or high blood pressure. For example, several of the antidepressant medications have been shown to decrease the frequency and severity of hot flashes. These medications have been discussed on page 45.

Remember that any hormonal treatment for hot flashes could affect breast cancer recurrence. This is particularly important because most of the hot flash studies have been conducted over weeks or months, rather than years. So we don't know what the long-term effects might be. Many of the herbal and plant estrogens, including soy, have estrogen-like properties and can't be assumed to be safe for breast cancer survivors. Once again, natural does not equal safe or free of risk. We become very concerned when we learn that our patients who are breast cancer survivors appropriately avoid prescribed estrogen but are loading up on soy products. Until more is known, this seems like a risky gamble, particularly for women with estrogen receptor positive tumors.

In addition to hot flashes, women may be troubled by vaginal dryness. For these symptoms, local estrogen, especially the estrogen ring, might be considered, since the ring delivers high concentrations of estrogen where it is needed, the vagina, but little into the bloodstream. And remember that there are other options to treat vaginal symptoms, including lubricants, moisturizers, and more sex.

The new reservations about long-term estrogen use for all women mean that much more attention is now being devoted to nonhormonal treatments, which may be of particular benefit to breast cancer survivors.

And Keep Your Eye on Breast Cancer Prevention

Watch for the results of the STAR (Study of Tamoxifen and Raloxifene) trial. This study will look at the effect of tamoxifen and raloxifene on the prevention of breast cancer. It will therefore contribute new data that will be helpful in making treatment decisions.

Also look for the continued development of a new class of medication called aromatase inhibitors, including exemestane, letrozole, and anastrozole. These medications derail the production of estrogen at the chemical level and have promise in breast cancer prevention.

Preventing Ovarian Cancer

We've learned a huge amount about the genetics of breast cancer and ovarian cancer. And we are likely to learn more about women at the highest risk. Screening to detect early cancer will probably be refined over the next few years. Right now, however, genetic testing is not recommended for the average woman.

Some women have their ovaries removed in order to significantly reduce the risk of ovarian cancer. This is completely understandable for women who have completed their family histories and have discovered family members who have had breast or ovarian cancer and who also carry the gene.

For the average woman, however, the risk of ovarian cancer is tiny, less than 1 percent, so the wholesale removal of ovaries is not a good idea. And remember, any surgery carries risks. Nonetheless, the stories of the suffering and death of women like the gifted comedian Gilda Radner are terrifying. In the past, women who were at high risk for ovarian cancer were given ultrasounds of their ovaries, plus a blood test for a marker called CA125. However, this test was developed to monitor treatment for ovarian cancer once it was diagnosed, not for early identification. It also creates a number of false positives, leading to unnecessary anxiety and medical procedures. Also, an ultrasound can show only tumors of a certain size. So this combination is not as precise a screening procedure as we would like. The good news is that a blood test is being developed that we hope will allow the detection of ovarian cancer very early on. So be on the lookout for it.

Research Advisers

Some people give up on making sense of the monumental amount of Internet information and turn to research advisers. These companies will, for a fee, gather and distill information about a specific problem. Some of them will also identify clinical trials. Some sites have been founded by patients, others by physicians and health care professionals, and still others by reference librarians. The sources currently available deal primarily with cancer.

The problem here is the variability of the credentials and the potential bias of the experts. Some services are indirectly funded by pharmaceutical companies. Many of the sites state that their goal is to synthesize available information and provide the consumer with maximum choice. Time will tell whether this option, which ranges in cost from $15 to $500, is both fair-minded and practical. In the meantime, a consistently reputable source of information about cancer treatments is the Web site www.cancer.org, run by the American Cancer Society.

CHAPTER SIX

○─○─○

Communicating with Your Doctor About Your Health

Are you nervous when you talk with your doctor? You are not alone—most people are, and that includes us. There is even a condition known as white-coat hypertension, a form of high blood pressure caused by anxiety in the doctor's office. Even though you are in the process of becoming your own menopause expert, you will likely feel nervous or uncomfortable with your doctor from time to time. This chapter will help you learn how to communicate more effectively with your doctor.

First, a note about terms: In general, we prefer to talk about health care professionals or clinicians rather than doctors, acknowledging that a comprehensive team achieves the best approach to health and that women see many different clinicians. The specific interactions we address in this chapter, however, are primarily those related to the patient-physician relationship. Most of the women we've met tend to be more upset by conversations with their physicians than by interactions with other health care professionals. We use the word *doctor* at times because that's the word that most patients use.

Research suggests that good communication is one of the top three competencies most patients value in their doctors. Yet at the same time, poor communication is an all-too-common complaint. We hear stories of miscommunication on almost a daily basis. There are many reasons for these problems.

Dr. Aaron Lazare, a professor of psychiatry at the University of Massachusetts, suggests that patients routinely feel shame and humiliation in medical interactions. No wonder. You are usually visiting a doctor because you are suffering from pain or discomfort or you need information or medication. Thus you are in a classic one-down position. Doctors also have advanced degrees and professional status, which reinforces their authority. Lazare also adds that the act of disrobing in a sterile, uncomfortable examining room and the exposure of your body to a stranger when you are in psychological or physical pain are inherently humiliating and create feelings of vulnerability. Thus, merely being a patient can make communication difficult.

There are additional barriers to good communication. Although many more women have entered medicine, a gender differential still exists with many female patients seeing male doctors. You may feel more uncomfortable if your doctor is much older or younger than you are, or if he or she is from a different cultural background. Some lesbians are uncertain as to whether, when, and how to come out to their doctors. For example, one of our lesbian patients answered an intake questionnaire responding that she was in a sexual relationship but noted that she did not need birth control information. She wondered why her doctor didn't follow up on that seemingly contradictory statement. From our experience in teaching physicians, we know that they are sometimes uneasy asking questions about sexuality, whether out of concern for the patient's privacy or out of their own discomfort with the issue.

As patients, then, we have anxieties and concerns about our health and relationships with our doctors. From the doctor's perspective, there are a lot of issues, too. The average primary care physician cares for a total of 2,500 patients. In a forty-year career, he or she will have 120,000 to 160,000 encounters with patients. And now the corporate takeover of health care has led to increased time pressures. All of this has resulted in major stress on the doctor-patient relationship. Both patients and doctors are frustrated. One study found that doctors interrupt their patients, on average, seventeen *seconds* into the interview.

Other research revealed that the typical patient asks only an average of four questions during a fifteen-minute interview. And remember, this includes questions about prescribed medications.

Even reaching a doctor by phone can be frustrating. The TV commentator Andy Rooney recently showed a collection of prescription medications marketed directly to patients. All of them included the phrase "talk to your doctor." He then proceeded to call his doctor, only to confront one of those voice mail from hell systems. He gave up.

Some patients are using e-mail messaging with their doctors. The success of this really depends on your physician's comfort with e-mail communication. Some physicians do not want to use it, while others welcome the opportunity to answer questions when they have the time to do so.

Medical technology is a mixed blessing, too. Edward Shorter, Ph.D., is professor in the history of medicine at the University of Toronto. He has written several fascinating books, including *History of Psychiatry* and *The Health Century*. In his book *Doctors and Their Patients: A Social History*, Shorter traced the history of doctor-patient communication and suggested that doctors paid more attention to the patient's story before the development of antibiotics—sulfa drugs in the 1930s and penicillin in the 1940s. Thus, Shorter noted, by the late 1940s, medicine became a war between the doctors and the microbes, leaving the patient out. "Battle lines were drawn between doctor and aberrant molecules, with patients left on the sidelines. A new technology had intervened."

Similarly today, with the availabilities of high-tech MRIs, CAT scans, and other diagnostic procedures, there is even more of a movement away from spending time with patients. Some call it "high tech, low touch," to indicate that doctors send patients for tests rather than examining them.

The menopause question has become similarly complex. Women went through hot flashes without medication until Premarin was introduced in 1942. Until very recently and still too often today, physicians reduce a woman's entire midlife experience to "estrogen—yes or no?" Yet we now have an array of other options for treating the symptoms of menopause and preventing the conditions associated with it. Therefore, conversations need to be longer and more detailed.

Of course we wouldn't want to return to the preantibiotic age. It is good news that we have so many medications, diagnostic tests, and other options for treating the symptoms and associated conditions of menopause. But it is a challenge to obtain adequate information and to discuss options in this situation.

Establishing Good Communication with Your Doctor

The process of establishing and maintaining good communication with your doctor is just that—a process, not a onetime conversation. It may have its ups and downs, but there is a lot you can do to foster an open dialogue.

The first issue is understanding that you have the right to adequate discussion of your health. Try to get over your concern about bothering your doctor. Many women don't feel entitled to ask detailed questions, especially if their doctors are male. Then again, we have heard some patients say the same thing about female doctors, adding, "She must be so busy, with her practice and her family." It doesn't matter. Patient education is a critically important aspect of health care. You have a right—actually, a duty to yourself—to become informed.

To begin, if you need a new primary care doctor or want to change doctors, ask friends and colleagues for recommendations. Doctors have reputations for being good communicators, so you'll know from the beginning that the person values patient education. But be forewarned, some of the best communicators also tend to run late. You can solve this problem by checking in with the office the day of your appointment and see how the schedule is going. Alternatively, bring something along to keep you busy—catch up on your correspondence or read that book you've been waiting to finish.

Once you've gotten a doctor who values communication, the next step is to understand your own need for information. Are you a medical information junkie? Do you like to know all the details of your options or do you want just the big picture? Some researchers suggest that there are two major categories of patients: repressors and sensitizers. Repressors (avoiders) tend to cope with medical stress by not thinking about it or by distracting themselves. These patients do not appear to be anxious. Sensitizers, on the other hand, are anxious and handle the anxiety by gathering information and by paying careful attention to details. You probably already know which kind of patient you are: If you are a repressor, you might want a small amount of general information, and if you are a sensitizer, you'll want more detail. But your physician won't know how much information you want unless you communicate your needs in this area.

It's sometimes difficult for doctors to gauge their patients' level of interest or understanding of medical information, and you may feel as if they talk down to you. Again, be as clear and straightforward as possible. For example, you might say, "It's not that I don't understand *why* I need to lose weight, it is just extremely difficult for me to do." This type of readjustment can often be effective. If you find that you feel talked down to consistently over time, however, your doctor may not be a good match for you.

Some doctors go too far in the other direction, overloading you with information without giving a specific recommendation. This may be an overreaction to the consumer movement in health care, which advocates that patients be informed of all of their treatment options. As much as we support this philosophy, physicians need to offer more than a list of choices. It's appropriate to discuss the research on each medical option and leave the final decision up to the patient, but the physician should also offer a recommendation. After all, he or she is a professional with expertise. Too often—possibly because of a misguided reaction to patients' rights, fear of litigation, time pressure, or a lack of communication skills—a physician will omit the recommendation or bury it in detail that is unclear.

It can be helpful to ask a very direct question: "What would you recommend if I were your sister [wife, daughter, or other family member] and in this situation?" Most of them will be happy to respond to this question with their best judgment. (Even if your physician is a woman, use the family member question. Asking her what she herself would do is a bit too direct and might feel like an invasion of her privacy.)

If your doctor is reluctant, try again. "I think I understand my choices, but given all of them, what is your best judgment? I value your opinion and I'd like to consider it in making my decision." This part of the dialogue restates your interest in knowing his/her professional opinion but also reasserts that you will make your own decision. It's best to do this at the beginning of the appointment so your doctor is forewarned and can plan the visit accordingly.

Organize your questions and concerns. If you have a good memory and don't get anxious, you can be prepared mentally. Otherwise, take notes. You might also keep a diary of your symptoms for a few days. That way you'll be able to answer questions about, for example, sleep disruption, hot flashes, and mood changes.

You might also call ahead and inform the staff that you'd like to discuss treatment options with the doctor. They can schedule you accordingly. If there has been any miscommunication when you get to the office, restate the purpose of your appointment. Again, be clear. If you are asking for *initial* information about menopause, say so. Some offices encourage a dialogue with a nurse or health educator before you see the physician.

Now that you understand your general needs, you should also consider your goals for each office visit. The clearer you are, the more likely you are to have your needs met. For example, are you trying to gather initial information or have you made some tentative decisions that you want to discuss? Let your doctor know.

At the end of a visit, your physician should summarize what's been said, but alas, that often does not occur. So you can do it. For example, you can say, "So that I understand you, I should take the new medication twice a day for ten days and then call you. And I'll also schedule my mammogram." This gives your doctor a chance to clarify if there is any confusion.

This brings us to another major concern. Many office visits consist of little more than a physician handing over a prescription. At our Menopause Town Meetings, many women tell us they are taking medications without knowing why. One of the most common examples is the use of low-dose contraceptives for perimenopausal women. A woman usually says something like "I'm taking a low-dose oral contraceptive because my periods were irregular." But then when we ask "Did it *bother* you that your periods were irregular?" she says, "No." So what went wrong? Most likely, one of two things. First, many physicians are pragmatic and action-oriented. They want to help and interpret help-ing as *doing* something—writing a prescription or ordering a test. In fact, one of the maxims we use when teaching communication skills to young physicians is "Don't just do something, sit there!" So when the physician heard that a woman had irregular periods, he or she assumed that this was a symptom worth treating. Indeed, low-dose oral contra-ceptives will regulate menstrual cycles.

Another possibility is that the physician wasn't paying careful attention and was on autopilot. Perhaps so many patients have requested low-dose oral contraceptives that it has become the norm, or the physician believes that this is a good general practice. You can interrupt this process by responding, "But the periods don't bother me."

The Process of Being Assertive

We think of being assertive as something like standing up for our rights. But in reality it is a series of steps. First, you need to state your thoughts and feelings, or summarize something that has happened. Then you need to say what you want to happen. Many of us can pass the first assertiveness test, which is stating our concerns. Yet when we meet with some resistance, we retreat. Here is a common scenario:

> **Joan:** Doctor, I've been thinking, and I'd like to try vitamin E to help with hot flashes.
>
> **Doctor:** Why do that? Estrogen is much better. Here is a prescrip-tion.
>
> *Joan retreats.*

Even though physicians may be less enthusiastic about hormones these days, this scenario is still common. In any case, Joan needs to try again:

> **Doctor:** Here is a prescription.
>
> **Joan:** Thanks, but I have some concerns about estrogen, so I'd like to try vitamin E instead.

Doctor: I think you're overreacting.

The physician hands Joan the prescription. Joan retreats.

Joan has restated her decision only to be accused of overreacting, a word often used to disarm a person during a disagreement. So let's try it one more time:

Joan: That may be, but I've thought this through and I hope you'll respect my decision.

Note that Joan did not address the possibly offensive word *overreacting*. It wasn't necessary during this conversation, though it might be at another time. In this situation, Joan consistently stated her opinion and indicated that she wished to be respected.

On the other hand, Joan's doctor might have wanted to emphasize the effectiveness of estrogen and then Joan could share her concerns about it. Then, in the spirit of communication and respecting her physician's expertise, a more detailed conversation might have followed. If that was the intention, the physician could have said, "I think estrogen is still the best choice. Before you make a decision about vitamin E, let's talk about it." Or "Why don't we see how it goes with vitamin E and then reevaluate?"

Nonverbal communication is another key factor in being assertive. Your mother was right: Sit up straight, look 'em in the eye, and speak clearly. Avoid having the discussion when you're in a particularly vulnerable situation, like while having your Pap smear. Yes, we've heard from many women that their important conversations take place *during* an internal exam or breast exam. Not exactly a comfortable time to think through a decision.

You can notice your doctor's nonverbal communications, too. Some doctors unconsciously use dismissive gestures. These often occur in discussions about complementary, alternative, or any controversial therapies. The two most common are the shrug or the slight sweep of the hand, often paired with "I don't know about that." While the verbal statement may be true, combining it with the shrug or the hand wave communicates a lack of interest or dismissiveness.

In that case, you have at least two choices. You can ignore it and forge ahead, restating your interest in, say, acupuncture as a treatment for hot flashes, or you can respond, adding, "Well, I hope you'll be open to this. Here is an article I read." You could also ask your physician to speak to another health care professional. Or "Dr. Smith, the acupuncture specialist would be happy to talk to you." This is usually true. Professionals from the complementary or alternative disciplines are usually eager to collaborate with physicians.

If you are extremely anxious or this is a major decision, such as whether to have a hysterectomy, take your spouse/partner or a friend with you. The other person may remember a question (or answer) you forget. You can share your reactions after the appointment.

Difficult Conversations

Some symptoms are more difficult to discuss than others, especially those related to sex. We've also found that many women are mortified to talk about incontinence. No wonder, since it is the focus of jokes about elderly women and some demeaning television commercials. But try to remember that your physician has probably heard whatever you have to say many times before. Even though you may feel embarrassed, try to put it on the agenda right away.

> **Doctor**: Miranda, you look well. How are you doing?
>
> **Miranda**: Not too well actually, Doctor. I want to talk about hot flashes and the pain I have during intercourse.

Try to avoid the "doorknob" comment or question, when you are on your way out the door. Many times we're anxious or embarrassed, so we leave something until the end of the appointment. This is understandable, but a bad idea. Doctors hate doorknob comments, especially when they contain important information. They want to allocate the time in an appointment to help you, and they can't if they don't know your agenda early on. You won't have optimal communication when you've surprised your doctor with a new symptom or major concern.

Of course doorknob comments go both ways. We recently spoke

to a woman who was trying to decide whether to have a hysterectomy. As she asked some questions, the doctor stood up and put his hand on the doorknob, answering quickly. Undeterred, the woman kept asking. Now he opened the door, so she stopped. We suggested that she say, "I can see that you need to leave now. When would be a good time for you to answer these questions?"

Suppose you want to bring up a difficult topic like depression or sexual abuse. You are most likely to get the best treatment if you are direct and open with your physician or health care professional. Physicians are human, however; they sometimes make mistakes or may not be as sensitive as we would like them to be. For example, let's say you have been waiting for your physician for over half an hour. He or she comes into the examining room and in a hurried fashion apologizes but seems preoccupied. You try to bring up your issue of depression, but you feel brushed off, or minimized. Be as direct as possible; state, "I'm concerned that I've been depressed." Sometimes physicians, in their attempt to be supportive, minimize problems and say something like "There is a lot of that these days." If this is the case, state again, ". . . but I know I'm having a problem here and I think I could use a referral to a psychotherapist."

No matter how hard we all try, sometimes interactions just don't go so well. If you're uncomfortable with the conversation, take some time. End the meeting. Think it over. Return to your other resources: a friend; a self-help group; a pharmacist; some other health care professional. If it is a disagreement, you can acknowledge the situation and add: "I'll think about it and what you said and hope that you'll do the same for me." Try again another time.

Extreme Situations

Most physicians try to communicate well with their patients. Still, if you have persistent problems with a physician's attitude, whether it is arrogance, an unwillingness to answer questions, or a consistent dismissal of your concerns, it's time to start looking for a new doctor. Your primary care doctor needs to be someone you respect and trust and in whom you can confide. Even if you are in an HMO or clinic setting, you have the right to switch doctors.

Unfortunately, there are a few problem individuals in every profession, including medicine. So if you feel extremely uncomfortable or unsafe with your physician, trust your instincts. If your boundaries have been violated by inappropriate physical contact or your doctor has breached confidentiality, you should switch. Any clearly inappropriate behavior should be reported to your state board of medical licensing. You have the right to a safe and trusting relationship.

The more actively involved you are in any health decision, the more likely you are to follow through. Keep these points in mind for your next appointment:

- Be prepared.
  —Know your goals for the visit.
  —List your questions.
  —Call ahead if you need a longer visit.

- Be clear.
  —State your goals at the beginning of the appointment.
  —Prioritize your concerns.

- Be assertive:
  —Ask direct questions.
  —Restate.
  —Summarize.

- Think ahead for the future.
  —Request a follow-up by phone, letter, or appointment.
  —Ask "what if" questions (e.g., "What if I find I can't tolerate the stomach upset with this medication?").

- Ask for more if you are not satisfied: another appointment; a referral to another health professional; or additional sources of information.

- Bring a family member or a friend.

Keep Your Eye On

Imagine this. You go to your doctor to talk about your menopause concerns. Rather than having a rushed discussion or being given a pamphlet, you are given an Internet address. At your leisure, you type in your concerns about symptoms and conditions, as well as your family and personal medical histories. You are also asked about your treatment preferences. Then, via the Internet, you and your doctor are given a report, based on the most up-to-date research, summarizing your concerns as well as your treatment options. At this point you and your doctor can have a fully informed discussion.

This technology will be available in the not-too-distant future. Dr. Nananda Col at Harvard Medical School has a federal grant to develop this system to facilitate communication about menopause between women and their doctors. We are assisting Dr. Col in developing accurate and understandable information. We will evaluate the decision-making process, especially women's comfort with the system and satisfaction with the shared decisions involved in menopausal health.

○─○─○

CHAPTER SEVEN

Making a Plan

We have now arrived at the stage for you to apply the knowledge you have gained. The planning stage of the Stages of Change Model we described in Chapter 4 is crucial. The more precise the plan, the better you will be able to evaluate it and make any necessary adjustments later on.

Any good plan relies on a thorough assessment of the problem. Try not to jump ahead to treatment choices. All too often we fall into the trap of reducing the options to "Hormone therapy—yes or no?" or "I'll use only natural solutions." It's fine to start out with certain values and preferences, but try to keep an open mind. By using an analysis of your concerns you can then move on to treatment choices with a clearer sense of your needs and priorities.

When you are taking stock of your concerns, you want to be aware of any family history of such diseases as breast cancer, endometrial and ovarian cancer, osteoporosis, colon cancer, heart disease, strokes, and Alzheimer's disease. For example, if you have a strong family history of breast cancer, you may want to avoid medications that further increase this risk and opt for medications shown to decrease the risk.

The following charts can help you evaluate your family

history and other risk factors for heart disease, osteoporosis, and breast cancer. These are not to be used for self-diagnosis. Each patient is different and you should use them for discussion with your own health care professional.

CHART 1

Am I at Risk for Heart Disease?

If you answer yes to any of the following questions, you are considered at risk for heart disease. The more that apply to you, the greater your risk.

	YES	NO
Do you smoke? (This remains the number one preventable heart disease risk factor for women.)	☐	☐
Do you have a family history of heart disease? (This refers to heart disease in your father or brother before age 55; or your mother or sister before 65)	☐	☐
Are you sedentary? (Sedentary people are nearly twice as likely to have heart disease than active people.)	☐	☐
Do you have diabetes? *(Diabetic women have twice the risk of heart disease.)*	☐	☐
Do you have high blood pressure?	☐	☐
Is your HDL cholesterol less than 40 or LDL greater than 130?	☐	☐
Are you overweight? (People who are 30 percent overweight or more are at a greater risk of heart disease.)	☐	☐

Source: Adapted from National Heart, Lung and Blood Institute, 2002.

CHART 2 ———————————————————————

Am I at Risk for Osteoporosis?

If you answer yes to any of the following questions, you are considered at risk for osteoporosis. The more that apply to you, the greater your risk.

	YES	NO
Are you white or Asian?	☐	☐
Do you have a family history of osteoporosis?	☐	☐
Are you slim?	☐	☐
Do you have a small frame?	☐	☐
Did you have early menopause (before age 40)?	☐	☐
Do you smoke?	☐	☐
Do you drink moderate or heavy amounts of alcohol (more than seven drinks per week)?	☐	☐
Are you overly sedentary?	☐	☐
Has your diet been low in calcium (less than 1,000 mg per day)?	☐	☐
Are you taking steroid medications or medications for thyroid disease, blood clots, or seizures?	☐	☐
Do you have a history of abnormal absence of menstrual period?	☐	☐
Do you have a history of anorexia nervosa?	☐	☐

Source: Adapted from National Heart, Lung and Blood Institute, 2002.

CHART 3

Am I at Risk for Breast Cancer?

If you answer yes to any of the following questions, you are considered at risk for breast cancer. The more that apply to you, the greater your risk.

	YES	NO
Do you have a family history of breast cancer? *(Women with a single first-degree relative with breast cancer of one breast have a small increase in risk. Women with a male family member with breast cancer, multiple first-degree relatives with breast cancer, or relatives with breast cancer of both breasts before menopause are at the greatest increased risk.)*	☐	☐
Did you start your menstrual period early (before age 12)?	☐	☐
Did you experience a late menopause (after age 55)?	☐	☐
No pregnancies, or was your first pregnancy after you were 30 years old?	☐	☐
Do you drink moderate or heavy amounts of alcohol (more than seven drinks a week)? *(Evidence suggests that there may a small increase in risk for women drinking more than a light amount of alcohol.)*	☐	☐
On mammograms, do you have dense breasts?	☐	☐

Source: Adapted from National Heart, Lung and Blood Institute, 2002.

In addition to family history and other risk factors, your own individual medical history is relevant. For example, if you have been taking thyroid hormone, you may be at greater risk for osteoporosis. Thus bone densitometry testing may be important in making your decisions. So record all of your medications on a chart similar to the one on page 112.

Prescription Medications

NAME	DOSAGE	REASON FOR TAKING	HOW LONG

Over-the-Counter Medications (ibuprofen, decongestants, etc.)

NAME	DOSAGE	REASON FOR TAKING	HOW LONG

Herbal Preparations

NAME	DOSAGE	REASON FOR TAKING	HOW LONG

Symptoms

The most common symptoms in the early stages of perimenopause and menopause are hot flashes, night sweats, and sleep disturbance. Many women also complain of mood changes, especially unexplained sadness or rapid changes in emotions. About five years after menopause, 25 percent of women experience vaginal dryness. And 15 to 35 percent of women over the age of 60 have problems with incontinence.

Hot Flashes

There is a lot of variation in women's experiences of hot flashes. Although most women report hot flashes during the menopausal transition, not all of them interfere with daily life. Studies suggest that from 75 to 85 percent of menopausal women are in the same boat. Still, about 15 percent of women state that hot flashes are severe.

If you want to see how your hot flashes are affecting you, use your hot flash diary to record your experiences. Record the severity (1 = just noticeable; 3 = the worst!). Also, watch for triggers (spicy foods, coffee, alcohol, stress). It might be easiest to fill in your diary at the end of the day. In the morning you can record your night sweats.

Mood Swings and Quality of Life

"I've just been down for no reason lately," or "One minute I'm fine and the next I'm crying or irritable in response to the least little thing." These are the two most common types of midlife mood problems. The issue of mood swings during the menopausal years is a somewhat controversial topic. Once again, a good assessment can help sort out your mood.

You can use a mood diary in a similar way to your hot flash diary, recording any rapid mood changes as well as an overall daily score. For example, you may have one or two episodes in a day when you feel intensely sad or angry (use a 1 to 5 scale). But overall you felt pretty good (a 3, with 1 = extremely sad and 5 = happy). Try to do this for a few weeks to see if there is a general pattern.

In addition, review your medical history, and your family history. Have you had feelings like this before? Did you ever take medication for depression? Do your moods now feel the way they did before? Has anyone else in your family had mood problems, depression, problems with alcohol? We ask you all these questions not to annoy you, but because these answers are important to creating the best plan. For example, if you have a family history of clinical depression, you are at greater risk. Similarly, if you have been treated for depression before, it can recur.

Three Women's Stories

Terry

Let's see how our assessment works with Terry, a 52-year-old elementary school teacher. Terry is a funny, irreverent, energetic woman who has been married to Bill for 25 years; they have two teenage boys. Casually dressed, she jokes a lot, even when discussing her menopause. She came to see us complaining of frequent hot flashes. She didn't mind them too much because she wore layers of clothing that she could easily shed in the classroom. However, recently she was beginning to feel down and somewhat irritable. She was still able to enjoy teaching, but with teenage sons, she felt frayed at home. "And it's not just the boys. Sure, they are noisy and demanding at times, but I'm usually fine. Now—well, I'm just not myself." Her last period was almost a year ago.

Terry filled out a hot flash diary and mood diary. These indicated seven to eight hot flashes per day, but they were short, with an intensity of 2. More important, although Terry wasn't sure, she thought she had many night sweats and remembers a lot of tossing and sheets ripping off. She also told us that she was tired a great deal of the time.

Assessment: Terry has a somewhat typical menopausal pattern of symptoms. Her main concerns were hot flashes and mood changes. Terry had gone almost a full year without a period. She could have had a blood test to check her FSH, but there was really no need, since Terry was clearly experiencing menopausal hot flashes and night sweats.

So we opted to target the hot flashes for treatment. To be more precise, we targeted night sweats because Terry felt that she could tolerate the hot flashes, but the disruption in her sleep was bothersome.

Turning to the mood swings, Terry felt somewhat down and tired. She had bursts of irritability or sadness, about two to three times a week—not too often, but more often than she considered normal. Terry had no previous history of depression. In addition, she was able to remember that she'd been having hot flashes for well over a year and had become moody and tired just a few months ago. This pattern of mood changes associated with the hot flashes and night sweats is quite common. Sleep disruption has been implicated as one possible cause of depressed mood during menopause.

We also looked at the other symptoms of major depression and of chronic low-grade depressed mood, or dysthymia. We saw that Terry was not hopeless, nor had she lost or gained weight or felt unable to concentrate. In contrast to the negativism seen so often in depression, Terry tended to be an optimistic, cheerful woman. So Terry did not have a major depression or dysthymia. Thus far, we had targeted hot flashes and night sweats. We also assumed that if we did so and improved her sleep, Terry's mood might improve.

Prevention: There are many conditions associated with getting older that we want to prevent, including osteoporosis, cancer, and heart disease. The average 50-year-old woman has a 31 percent lifetime chance of death from ischemic heart disease, a 2.8 percent risk of death from breast cancer, a 2.8 percent risk from a osteoporotic hip fracture, and a 0.7 percent risk from endometrial cancer. So heart disease is the number one killer of women. But then again, none of us is the average woman. Each one of us has a unique family history and group of symptoms and long-term concerns that should be considered.

In Terry's family, her parents were still alive at age 82. Her father had some high blood pressure, now controlled with medication. However, Terry's mother had a slight dowager's hump, a curvature that results from spinal fractures. Her grandmother and great-aunts also had osteoporosis. So one of Terry's major concerns was preventing osteoporosis.

Osteoporosis is the thinning of the bones or low bone mass that occurs from the deterioration of the internal structure of the bone. The condition leads to bone fragility and fractures. The lifetime risk for a 50-year-old woman for a hip fracture is 16 percent, 15 percent for a wrist fracture, and 32 percent for a fracture of the vertebrae. Terry knew that her grandmother had died in a nursing home after breaking her hip and developing pneumonia.

With respect to prevention, we wanted to be sure that Terry's lifestyle would help maintain her bone mass. She did exercise three times a week on a treadmill. This was great for maintaining bone strength in her legs, but it wasn't helping the bones in her arms. So we suggested that she add two sessions a week of upper body strength training with free weights, a rowing machine, or a racket sport.

Terry was a good candidate for a bone density test. A slight woman from a Scandinavian background, with osteoporosis in her family, she wanted to know whether she exhibited any early signs of osteoporosis. Most insurance plans cover the cost of a bone density test, which is similar to an X-ray and causes no discomfort.

Terry's results did reveal osteopenia, or some early thinning of the bone. These results were discouraging to Terry, who was determined to prevent osteoporosis. We wanted to give Terry a wide range of choices in order to help her prevent this potentially debilitating condition.

Fortunately, Terry didn't smoke or take any medications associated with osteoporosis. She wasn't taking enough calcium, though, given the recommendation of 1,200 to 1,500 milligrams per day for postmenopausal women. Terry was only consuming about 1,000 milligrams, since she took one 500-milligram supplement but consumed very few dairy products or other foods high in calcium. Her supplement did contain the necessary 400 to 800 IU of vitamin D needed to properly absorb calcium.

Terry's blood pressure was 120/80, her cholesterol was 180, and since she went to the gym three times a week to use the treadmill, she was not concerned about heart disease at this point. She felt that she was doing all that she could.

Terry had also seen two friends suffer with breast cancer. Although her grandfather had died of pancreatic cancer, breast cancer was not in her family. Still, Terry had worries about taking estrogen. She was aware of some studies linking estrogen to an increased risk of breast cancer.

So in summary, Terry's chief concerns were her vasomotor symptoms—hot flashes and night sweats—and her mood problem, along with her desire to prevent osteoporosis and avoid an increased risk of breast cancer. At one point in time, hormone therapy would have been the perfect short- and long-term choice for Terry. On a short-term basis, it is by far the most effective treatment for hot flashes and night sweats. One study of women with hot flashes and depressive symptoms found that women placed on hormone therapy had improvement on scores for their emotions. Since Terry still had her uterus, her treatment would need to be estrogen with added progestin therapy, or EPT. This is necessary because early studies revealed that estrogen given alone could lead to endometrial cancer. By adding a progestin, the added risk for endometrial cancer is virtually eliminated. Terry could take progestin two weeks a month and have her periods return or she could take a smaller dose of progestin every day.

Today, hormone therapy might still be an option for treating Terry's hot flashes and night sweats on a short-term basis. However, there is currently a lot of debate and controversy about what constitutes short-term treatment with hormone therapy. The WHI results have taught us that there is, in fact, no absolutely safe duration. The increases in blood clots and heart attacks occurred within a year of starting combined hormone therapy. Similarly, the increased rate of abnormal mammograms was seen within a year. Although the additional breast cancer was not seen until four years into treatment, it was troubling that the cancers, when diagnosed, were at a later stage. Even though Terry knew that her individual risk of developing breast cancer was small, her risk of having an abnormal mammogram was high (about 1 in 25 women treated with EPT for one year). She did not want the anxiety and stress associated with an abnormal mammogram and what might follow.

With respect to her father's pancreatic cancer, we explained, that estrogen has *not* been shown to add to the risk of getting pancreatic cancer. Terry was surprised to learn this.

Terry had another possible plan: to first treat her hot flashes without any medication. By using her hot flash diary, she was able to identify two clear triggers: coffee and alcohol. So, she decided to eliminate these triggers first.

In addition, vitamin E has helped some people with hot flashes, even though on the whole, it is considered only marginally effective. The good news is that in appropriate doses, it has no downside. So now that Terry had noticed that there was only 60 IU of vitamin E in her daily multivitamin, she increased her dose to 800 IU per day. These two interventions, avoiding hot flash triggers and adding vitamin E, were Terry's initial choice for a treatment plan.

Cheryl

Cheryl's agenda was clear when she began her appointment. "Take me off of this stuff!" Her primary care doctor had prescribed a combination of estrogen and MPA (Prempro) five years ago when she was 52. At that time, many people believed that hormone therapy could protect women from heart disease.

Cheryl's doctor had good reasons to be concerned that she might develop heart disease. Cheryl was 30 pounds overweight. Five years earlier she had had an elevated cholesterol level, with her LDL far exceeding the desirable level of less than 130. However, she had declined to take medication for lowering cholesterol. Cheryl also had borderline hypertension, 130/85. She was a director of a busy nonprofit agency and rarely exercised.

Then Cheryl heard the reports on the radio: Not only was the Prempro *not* preventing the development of heart disease, it could actually *lead* to heart attacks and strokes in some women, and after four years was associated with breast cancer. She was so angry with her doctor that she didn't call her. Then she made an appointment in our practice. Fortunately, Cheryl didn't stop her Prempro suddenly. Many of the women who do have quite an unpleasant, intense resurgence of hot flashes.

Our first goal with Cheryl was reassurance. The good news was that she'd been on Prempro for only five years. Her heart risk factors had not worsened and she had not had a stroke or any cardiac symptoms. Her last mammogram was normal. Although she didn't do a breast self-exam every month, Cheryl said, "I sure did one the last two months after that news."

Cheryl's concern was completely valid. She had been taking Prempro for prevention—that is, to reduce her risk of heart disease. But we added that her doctor was neither careless nor misinformed. It is unfortunate that a study such as the Women's Health Initiative was not done before 1997, but doctors were working with the only data they had. Because of the earlier observational studies many women were prescribed estrogen to reduce the risk of heart disease.

At the same time we could now help her discontinue her Prempro and create a new plan. Cheryl had not experienced a lot of discomfort from hot flashes at the time of menopause. Since Cheryl was already diagnosed with elevated cholesterol, we reviewed lifestyle changes that would reduce her heart risk factors and improve her overall health.

Many of us groan when we hear the words *lifestyle change,* and think, "Great. Deprivation or exercise. And I already have no time." Yet the power of lifestyle change is enormous. If Cheryl lost some weight, just 10 pounds, she would reduce her risk of a heart attack by 33 to 55 percent. If she just became physically active rather than remain sedentary, she could reduce her risk by 45 percent. If she reduced her cholesterol, even by 10 percent, she'd reduce her risk by 20 to 30 percent. Fortunately, Cheryl had never smoked cigarettes, but if she had, quitting would reduce heart attack risk by 50 to 70 percent in five years. In fact, the result of the well-known Nurses' Health Study concluded that a full 82 *percent* of coronary heart disease events were a result of changeable lifestyle behaviors.

Faced with these impressive numbers, Cheryl wanted to try. She added, though, "Still, it is *so* hard." And, we know that this is true. Cheryl had many home and work responsibilities. In addition to having a responsible job that also involved evening meetings for advocacy work, Cheryl took care of her grandchildren on Saturdays to help her daughter, who was divorced. Although Cheryl's husband Matt, who also worked more than full-time as a contractor, shared the housework, life was still too busy. And as an advocate, she was a leader in the African American community. She was often called to help people. Cheryl enjoyed her life, but it was busy.

Using our knowledge of behavior change and Cheryl's concerns, she chose two distinct goals. She would start to reduce the fat in her diet and increase her physical activity. We helped Cheryl restructure her environment. The Stages of Change Model and related research suggests that this environmental planning would improve her chances of success.

Cheryl could identify her food issues quite well. She and her husband did not eat high-fat food most of the time. However, they often added butter to vegetables and Cheryl used cream in her four cups of coffee. "Okay, no butter on vegetables and milk in my coffee instead of cream."

In addition, as a working couple, Cheryl and Matt would eat out twice a week. Sometimes they'd go alone, and at other times, they'd take their daughter or grandchildren. Recently, public awareness has grown that the "supersize" and high-fat phenomenon not only affects fast-food restaurants but most restaurants. Portions are often double, even triple what a "normal" portion would be. So, we suggested a range of possibilities, from eating more salads (going easy on the dressing) to changing restaurants and especially avoiding french fries at fast-food restaurants. At other restaurants, Cheryl and her husband could share an entrée or order a grilled appetizer or salad.

With respect to exercise, like many Americans, Cheryl was sleep deprived and tired most of the time. "No way" was she going to go to the gym at 6 A.M. before work. We looked at her weekly schedule. We saw that she indeed had very little free time. This is when we suggested a two-fer—that is, accomplishing two goals with one behavior change. Cheryl attended an informal gathering of other administrators of non-profit agencies once a week. Most of these women were similarly stressed, midlife women with too little time and multiple responsibilities. So we asked Cheryl to inquire if the other women wanted to walk and talk. They readily agreed. Thus, they could get support and physical activity together. Cheryl and her husband also decided to walk for an hour, two other times during the week.

When Cheryl took care of her 7- and 5-year-old grandchildren, we suggested that they go out to a park whenever possible. Another two-fer, helping her daughter and getting exercise. This became a three-fer when Cheryl noticed that Darryl and Lauren were much more able to play quietly after they burned off some steam!

We agreed to reevaluate the plan after eight weeks. This reevaluation is based on the idea that long-term behaviors, such as eating a high-fat diet and remaining sedentary, are extremely difficult habits to change. If Cheryl did well, we could reinforce and support her changes. If, on the other hand, she had some difficulties, we could help her alter her plan.

Veronica

Veronica just couldn't seem to get going. She wondered, "Could it be menopause?" Veronica was 47, a successful banker, and in a committed long-term relationship with Sybil. Over the past four months Veronica had grown irritable and would wake up at 2 A.M. and not be able to get back to sleep. Her periods were irregular and she had a few hot flashes, but like many women, she was not terribly bothered by these. Still, she had started taking a low-dose birth control pill to regulate her cycles, which had become a total nuisance.

When we questioned Veronica more closely, we discovered that she also was pessimistic and negative most of the time and felt like a failure despite her good relationship and measurable success at work. Through tears, Veronica added, "I even have passing thoughts of suicide, for no good reason." Sybil was frightened of Veronica's deteriorating mood.

Veronica was not anemic and did not have a thyroid disorder, just to list two "mood culprit" medical conditions that can create symptoms of depression. We did wonder about the oral contraceptives, though, because they can cause mood problems.

Veronica's situation was a bit complicated. Her symptoms, at least the sadness and change in energy, could perhaps be traced back to the new medication. Veronica wasn't sure, however, especially since she been depressed twice before, the first time in her teens.

As a child, Veronica had had extremely critical and demanding parents. In retrospect, Veronica believed that her father had been a high-functioning alcoholic. He never missed work but came home every night to two cocktails, then wine with dinner. Veronica's mother, an artist, would periodically complain about her husband to her children but never directly addressed his drinking. And the parents' rocky marriage left little emotional energy for the children. As he grew older, Veronica's father became a severe alcoholic, drunk a great deal of the time.

Veronica believed that her first depressive episode was a reaction to the family dynamics. In addition, like many teenagers who identify themselves as somehow different, she was uncomfortable because she was a lesbian. Although she had not experienced much harassment, she was teased about being "such a jock." "Yeah," Veronica added, "it was code for lesbian."

A year of psychotherapy had helped Veronica separate herself in a positive way from her family when she went to college, but she became depressed again years later after a lover broke up with her.

Given her current depression, Veronica had several options. We could stop the low-dose birth control pill and see if her mood improved. If she didn't feel a lot better, then we could add psychotherapy and an antidepressant medication.

Since Veronica had had two previous episodes of depression, it is possible that perimenopause precipitated a third. However, the oral contraceptive seemed to increase her depressive symptoms and worsen her mood. This is the paradox for women who have had reproductive-related depressive episodes. As you remember, the hormone used to treat hot flashes, estrogen, needs to be combined with a progestin for women who still have their uterus. This is necessary in order to prevent endometrial hyperplasia, which can lead to uterine cancer. However, many of these same women find that the mood symptoms worsen when they take any form of progestin. They may have a similar response to low-dose contraceptives.

Fortunately, recent research, as detailed in Chapter 3, reveals that certain antidepressants can reduce hot flashes and treat symptoms of depression. These include venlafaxine (Effexor) and paroxetine (Paxil). So Veronica had other options.

Veronica tentatively decided to discontinue the oral contraceptive, and then later perhaps add an antidepressant. We recommended either 75 milligrams of venlafaxine or 20 milligrams of paroxetine per day because they had the added benefit of treating hot flashes and night sweats.

Veronica's story is important for another reason. Even if her menstrual history isn't taken into account, Veronica meets the criteria for a major depressive episode. She had lost sleep, didn't feel like eating, and couldn't concentrate well. Unlike Terry, Veronica was plagued by a profound and pervasive sense of sadness, to the point that she felt suicidal at times. "I wouldn't do it, though," she added.

Depression affects 10 to 20 percent of American women at any time. It tends to be underdiagnosed and undertreated. This is tragic because psychotherapy and antidepressant medication can successfully treat depression in most cases. But Veronica first wanted to stop taking oral contraceptives and see how she was doing. We arranged to see Veronica within two weeks in order to monitor her mood carefully, and also contracted with her to call us if her suicidal thoughts increased.

The Decision to Stay on Hormone Therapy

When some of the dust settled after the reports of the results of the Women's Health Initiative, we began to hear the position contrary to Cheryl's. Many women want to stay on hormone therapy. Some of these women feel pressure from their families and friends, the news reports, and even their doctors to discontinue their estrogen regimen. A few of them are quite defiant with a "Hell, no. We won't go!" attitude.

Let's look at the decision. Most women were prescribed hormone therapy originally for menopausal symptoms: hot flashes and night sweats and/or genitourinary problems. Then when they felt better because the symptoms had been successfully treated, they wanted to stay on the hormone therapy. As we have explained previously, most physicians were in favor of this decision because estrogen does prevent osteoporosis and there was a belief that estrogen also prevented heart disease. Now that there is evidence to the contrary with respect to hormone therapy and heart disease, and with additional data pointing to an increased risk of breast cancer, the risk-benefit evaluation has changed. So currently most professional associations recommend that hormone therapy *not* be prescribed for preventive purposes.

But what if a woman feels that hormone therapy is necessary for a better quality of life? This is a matter of personal preference and an individual choice. So let's look again at quality of life. What are the possible elements involved? Perhaps a woman is concerned about the return of hot flashes, with the potential for disrupting her daily life and causing sleep disturbance. Or perhaps the estrogen was used to treat vaginal thinning and dryness or to prevent or treat osteoporosis. Estrogen does improve the quality of sleep for women with menopausal symptoms. In addition, estrogen in some cases helps stabilize mood in perimenopausal women or may augment antidepressant therapy.

For all these situations, an informed decision involves consideration of the risks of hormone therapy compared to the other options for treatment. The percent increases in adverse events (heart attacks, strokes, blood clots, breast cancer) are important. On the other hand, these percentage increases translate to seven more adverse heart events and eight additional cases of breast cancer for every 10,000 person-years of treatment. These data were enough to decide not to expose additional women in a study to these risks. But that's not the same evaluation as one woman deciding for herself. So each woman should make a unique decision based on her values, her needs, and an understanding of the risks and benefits after discussion with her health care professional.

If you have a strong family history of breast cancer or if you have breast cancer, it is now accepted that you really should avoid estrogen. In addition, if you have been diagnosed with heart disease or blood clots, you should avoid taking hormone therapy. You can refer to our section of treatment choices in Chapter 3. Otherwise, if we look at the potential uses of estrogen listed above and remember the material from Chapter 3, each symptom has an alternative treatment. So it might be worth attempting another treatment option before making the decision to remain on estrogen indefinitely.

But first, don't do what too many women did: stop taking estrogen suddenly. Working with your physician, taper it off, over a few weeks, to prevent the return of hot flashes. Then you can treat each symptom with another option. Use our diary system to evaluate the change. Then you have more data with which to make an informed decision.

Some women contend that they just feel better overall. That's fine, but still worth a medication holiday as an experiment. Since hot flashes and night sweats are the most disruptive, it is important to note that usually, if it's been a few years and if you decrease estrogen slowly, you can avoid a resurgence of hot flashes.

If you do decide to remain on hormone therapy, you might consider doing the following:

- Cut back to a lower dose. For example, studies suggest that osteoporosis can be prevented by less than half of what was once prescribed; .3 mg rather than .625 mg of conjugated equine estrogen.
- Similarly, if you are using estrogen, for example, for uro-genital symptoms, you might consider vaginal (creams, rings or tablets) rather than systemic use (pills or patches).
  In both of these situations you are limiting your overall exposure to estrogen.
- Vigilantly monitor your breast health. Do a monthly breast self-exam. Don't forget your annual mammogram. Make sure your doctor does a thorough breast exam every year even if you have had a normal mammogram.
- Limit alcohol to no more than 1 to 2 drinks per day.
- Exercise, exercise, exercise. Stay physically active in your daily life as well. Take the stairs. Don't park so close to the store. Walk instead of drive.
- Watch your cholesterol and blood pressure. Monitor them with your doctor on a regular basis.
- Eat a heart-healthy diet. You don't need to starve. Just lower the fat content. Replace animal fat with olive oil. Spice up your food and cut down on salt. Invest in one of the heart-healthy cookbooks.
- It is worth reconsidering your decision in the future. This is a good idea with so much new research appearing. If the risks are shown to be less or additional benefits identified, you might be reassured. On the other hand, if more risks are found, you may decide to stop.

After all, it is your decision. If you've thought through the risks and benefits, you should accept your decision.

Now Terry, Cheryl, and Veronica all had plans. You can follow the same process. After you've reviewed your family history and personal medical history, identify your goals. Consider both your present symptoms as well as conditions you want to prevent. Next, choose a treatment plan and structure your environment to help you stick to that plan. In the next chapter we'll help you evaluate the results.

CHAPTER EIGHT

Is the Plan Working?

You've done an assessment, identified your goals, brushed up on your treatment options, and talked to your doctor. It's time to put your plan into action, then step back and evaluate its effectiveness.

How Are Your Symptoms?

Many women begin a treatment for a menopausal symptom and then sit back: decision made, case closed. Life goes on and you continue to use the treatment—or maybe you stop for one reason or another. This is probably not the best strategy.

A more systematic approach is to take the plan you've worked out with your doctor and try it for four to six weeks. Keep recording your symptoms in your diary during this time.

At the end of the trial period, take a look at the information you've collected. You can even calculate pre-treatment and post-treatment scores. Let's look at Terry's hot flash/night sweat diary. Terry's diary revealed some good news: Her hot flashes had been reduced by about 50 percent. But Terry was still only getting about two hours of uninterrupted sleep a night, and her moods hadn't improved much. So she concluded that eliminating hot flash triggers and adding 800 IU of vitamin E had offered only limited improvement in her symptoms.

After thinking it over again, Terry decided to try hormone therapy. After six weeks on Premphase, a combination of conjugated equine estrogen and a progestin, her hot flashes were almost eliminated, going from an average of three to less than one per day. Even better news was that she slept seven hours a night, her usual before she hit perimenopause. Terry's mood diary revealed she was much less irritable. "I love my sleep," she sighed with a smile.

Could this have been the placebo effect that we discussed in Chapter 2? If a woman takes any treatment for hot flashes and has a positive expectation, then even a sugar pill, or placebo, can lead to a 20 to 30 percent reduction. This isn't usually a problem; why not accept some good news? (Unless of course you are spending an inordinate amount of money for a minimal gain.) In Terry's case, however, the improvement in her hot flashes and night sweats was so dramatic that she could be pretty confident that the change was not a result of the placebo effect.

If you are uncertain about the effect of your treatment plan, you might conduct your own mini-experiment: Try stopping the treatment for a while and then evaluating whether your symptoms return.

Side Effects

It would appear that Terry's implementation of HT was a great success. Well, not exactly. Terry originally took Premphase, which is estrogen plus progestin. She would take estrogen alone for 2 weeks and then 2 weeks of estrogen and medroxyprogesterone acetate (MPA), a type of progestin. The MPA caused Terry's periods to be lighter than before and very predictable.

The return of periods did not exactly fill Terry's heart with glee. "So we take away the *one* good thing about menopause, no more periods?" Even so, she had tentatively decided that the return of her periods was worth it. The only problem was that Terry's mood diary revealed that she felt great during the first two weeks, but crashed on the MPA.

She didn't feel irritable as she had before treatment, but she felt extremely sad, tired, and weepy. ("PMS, too?")

What to do? We discussed a number of choices. First, Terry could switch the type of regimen she was on, cyclical combined HT (referring to cycles of medication to mimic menstrual cycles) to continuous combined HT. In the continuous combined plan, a smaller dose of progestin is taken every day. Over time, this regimen leads to no menstrual bleeding. A second option would be to switch to unopposed estrogen—that is, estrogen taken alone. Since Terry still had her uterus, however, this would require periodic endometrial biopsies—taking a sampling from the lining of the uterus, the endometrium, with a small plastic catheter. While the procedure is performed on an outpatient basis and does not require local anesthesia, it can be a little painful and cause some cramping. The biopsy can determine whether the estrogen is causing endometrial hyperplasia, a buildup of cells in the uterine lining that may lead to cancer. In that case, a woman would need a D & C, or dilation and curettage, to remove the hyperplasia.

"That's simple," said Terry. "Absolutely not." Terry's justifiable concerns about cancer, combined with the nuisance and potential discomfort of the endometrial biopsy, helped her eliminate this option. Another choice would be to switch from HT entirely to another medication or herbs. But these also might create side effects and would be less effective in treating her hot flashes.

Terry opted for the continuous combined regimen of HT. For convenience, she also decided to switch to a combination estradiol/progestin patch, which looks like a round piece of plastic tape, about the size of a quarter. The HT is absorbed through the skin and the patch is replaced twice a week. Terry found that her hot flashes and night sweats were still virtually eliminated and her mood was good. She did have some spotting at first. However, she didn't mind wearing minipads and was pleased to hear that this irregular bleeding should stop within six months.

What About Prevention?

Terry's experimentation with HT to treat her symptoms took awhile, but was a success. What about her concerns about osteoporosis? As we know, at one point, HT would have been prescribed for long-term prevention. The current thinking of numerous professionals is different, as evidenced by this part of a special report in the journal *Women's Health in Primary Care:* "Postmenopausal women who are taking estrogen plus progestin for the relief of menopausal symptoms can be assured that their absolute risk of harmful side effects is small and that the short-term use of HT for that indication may still be appropriate. However, clinicians should no longer prescribe this therapy for long-term use."

We worked out a plan in which Terry would stay on HT for one to two years and then gradually taper the dose off, ultimately discontinuing the medication. Terry could then use her diaries again to reevaluate her progress.

What should Terry do to preserve bone mass after she discontinued HT? Well, the first thing would be to have another bone densitometry test. It is fortunate that we now have an accurate way to assess Terry's progress. If the test still shows osteopenia, she has several choices (see Chapter 4), including the medications alendronate, risedronate, and raloxifene. Of course, calcium, vitamin D, and exercise remain essential to any plan to prevent osteoporosis.

Terry thought that in the future the SERM raloxifene might be best for her. It could prevent and treat osteoporosis, reducing her risk for spinal fractures by an estimated 30 to 50 percent. In addition, a study of over 7,000 women, followed for over three years, revealed that women who took raloxifene had a reduced risk of developing breast cancer, another concern of Terry's. Like the estrogen, raloxifene also reduces the bad cholesterol (LDL), but unlike estrogen, it does not increase the good cholesterol (HDL).

Even though we wanted Terry to begin to think about her options, she was fortunate to be able to wait a couple of years before making her decision. The SERMs are relatively new medications and two more years could reveal more about their potential benefits and risks. For example, although the effect on the lipids, or fat in the blood, is positive, we don't know yet about the actual prevention of coronary disease. The other possible risks of SERMs are an increase in hot flashes and risk of a blood clot (venous thromboembolism).

Meanwhile, what about Cheryl?

Cheryl's goals were to discontinue HT and reduce her risk factors for developing heart disease. She had targeted increased exercise and decreased fat in her diet. Specifically, she had planned to walk with her colleagues, do more physical activity with her grandchildren, and cut back on fatty foods, especially in restaurants.

By using our knowledge of the Stages of Change Model and environmental planning, we suggested that Cheryl first choose a date to implement her plan. Next, she should stock up on any needed supplies before her change date. Since Cheryl's main food plan was avoidance of fast food, she did not need to purchase many new foods. Like most of us, she needed more fruits and vegetables on hand. She also needed to buy 2 percent milk to replace the cream in her coffee. She improved the flavor by adding spices to vegetables instead of butter.

Cheryl had a decent pair of walking shoes to start, but she decided to treat herself to a new silver-colored high-tech pair if she stayed with her program for six weeks. This helped motivate her and also reinforced her efforts in a relatively short amount of time. It was particularly helpful that the reward was based simply on her sticking to her plan, not on some other criterion like the number of pounds lost. Sticking to the plan was the main goal over the long run.

Cheryl's diary was also useful in monitoring her plan. One study of people trying to lose weight revealed that just recording what they ate led to a 5-pound weight loss in a month. Cheryl's diary revealed fat in her diet that she could eliminate. She had the two culprits common in many women's diets: cream in her coffee and salad dressing. Cheryl had already reduced her caffeine to two cups of coffee in the morning. At noon she switched to decaf. She drank an additional 3 cups of decaf with 2 tablespoons of cream in each cup, so her total daily amount was 10 tablespoons of cream. That's not only 400 calories but also 35 grams of fat. Remember, on a 1,500-calorie-per-day program, you should only be eating 65 grams of fat per day. Cheryl couldn't stand skim milk in her coffee ("that grayish look") but accepted 2 percent milk. This saved over 29 grams of fat per day and 240 calories a day—a small, but not insignificant change in calories in the long run—and the fat reduction was critically important.

Salad dressing can be a hidden source of fat. Many women go to a salad bar with the purest of intentions, load their plate with greens but then top it with 4 to 5 tablespoons of fat-laden dressing. Cheryl had wisely avoided mayonnaise-based dressings but was unaware that some "light" dressings still contained 10 grams of fat.

If decreased fat intake and weight control are your goals, we've included different weight plan resources at the end of the book, but one excellent volume is *Strong Women Stay Slim* by Miriam E. Nelson, Ph.D., with Sarah Wernick, Ph.D. Dr. Nelson is a professor of nutrition at Tufts University, and her book includes different food plans based on lifestyle and needs, including the "I'm very busy," "I'm always hungry," and the "I crave sweets" plans.

So Cheryl was able to cut out a lot of dietary fat as a result of accurate self-recording. Her diary revealed even more valuable information. For example, on stressful days, she would consume a quick fix of a doughnut, a pastry, or some other fat-filled sweet carbohydrate in the afternoon. So another challenge was either to reduce stress or to substitute another stress-reducing behavior.

Like many women trying to eat in a healthy manner, Cheryl was eating too little protein. Her morning meal was half a bagel with jam and coffee. Her noon meal was vegetable-based salad, now with just a little dressing. We pointed out that by the middle of the afternoon, she was both stressed and really hungry. This set her up for an unhealthy need for carbs, sugar, and fat. By adding some protein, turkey, or tofu on her salad and some low-fat cheese with her bagel, she would feel fuller and less hungry later on.

In addition, Cheryl needed some new stress reduction plan for the afternoon. She had learned deep breathing exercises in a stress management class. As with all such techniques, the key is to find and take the time to implement them in a busy day. Cheryl found that she could take a walk around the block on most days. During our damp, cold New England winters, when walking is not a lot of fun, she could close the door to her office, listen to some music for a few minutes, do some deep breathing, and sip her decaf. Cheryl was fortunate that her administrative assistant had been worried about her health (sisterhood *is* powerful) and would protect Cheryl during these rare quiet moments.

Thus her daily logs helped us eliminate barriers to Cheryl's success. We also suggested that after ten weeks of increased exercise and less fat, she have her cholesterol checked again. And since her husband also had high blood pressure, the couple had invested in a blood pressure cuff so they could take their blood pressure at home.

Cheryl found that her cholesterol was a bit lower after ten weeks. In addition, like most women, she couldn't help but weigh herself, and she found out she'd lost four pounds. That pleased her, but we didn't emphasize the weight loss because Cheryl had lost and regained many pounds over the years. We wanted to reinforce other healthful measures, such as her brisk walking three times a week ("I'm into it now"). Although she might not see initial results, we knew that if she walked at 3 to 4 miles per hour, she could reduce her risk of cardiovascular disease by almost 50 percent.

After about seven more weeks Cheryl had a slip: "Actually, more like a tumble—I went to Burger King twice and my local ice cream parlor, too." She regained two pounds quickly. We reminded Cheryl that change was a long process, involving periodic relapses, and that she could learn from each slip. In this case, the grandchildren had begged her to go to Burger King. She was frustrated, but after succumbing to please them, she helped herself to a Whopper (39 grams of fat, 680 calories, even without those supersize fries!). So rather than focus on the mistake, we saw that we needed to add another aspect to the plan. First, we rehearsed ways to set limits with the grandchildren. Then we came up with alternative food choices, even those available at fast-food restaurants (grilled chicken, salads). Cheryl knew that a long-term issue was to learn ways to cope that didn't involve high-fat foods.

The issue of the doctor-patient relationship is also important to Cheryl's story. Cheryl was well down the road to improving her heart health, her level of fitness, and her family's health as well. So she was feeling better and more self-confident about her general health and well-being. But there was a problem remaining—Cheryl's feelings about her original doctor who had prescribed hormone therapy for the prevention of heart disease. Cheryl felt like she had been a guinea pig and had been exposed to an unnecessarily increased risk of breast cancer *and* of heart disease.

Cheryl is not alone. At our Menopause Town Meetings we've heard similar comments ranging from confusion and dismay to anger. One woman wondered aloud how so many women could have been prescribed hormone therapy as a long-term preventive wonder drug when it was never approved by the Food and Drug Administration for that use.

The answers are not simple. The observational studies, such as the Nurses' Health Study we described, were very persuasive. Estrogen is a wonder drug for blasting hot flashes away. There may well be a belief in estrogen as a cosmetic anti-aging potion also. Many women (and doctors) believe that estrogen helps preserve skin and hair, although the evidence for this is shaky. Many menopause preparations use the letters *fem* in their names to emphasize a refeminizing property, and ads for such preparations almost always emphasize youth.

Finally, the pharmaceutical companies inundated consumers and health care professionals alike with a pro-hormone-therapy perspective. They've had enormous advertising and marketing budgets and used them effectively. No one actually stated that estrogen could prevent heart disease (they can't do that without FDA approval), but it was a common belief.

But how could Cheryl evaluate her health care? She needed to look at her larger history with her physician, not just one action of prescribing hormones over the long term. The National Breast Cancer Coalition Fund (NBCCF) publishes a *Guide to Quality Breast Cancer Care* (www.stopbreastcancer.org or 800-622-2838 for more information). The guide suggests values that are applicable to quality health care in general, not just to concerns about breast cancer. Its emphasis on understanding your symptoms and concerns and using evidence-based medicine to identify treatment choices is similar to ours.

The guide also notes some necessary elements in good health care—respect and being treated as a whole person. Respect involves being aware of your doctor's thinking process. We also emphasize the value of comprehensive care. All too often menopausal women are reduced to their reproductive organs. Thus, treatment also became a question of hormones—yes or no? Even the terminology reflects value. Hormone therapy, once called hormone replacement therapy (yes, even by us in our earlier book), implies that of course a woman would want to replace her waning hormones, but as we've learned, maybe not. In contrast, comprehensive care attends to the whole person. With respect to menopause, hormones do play a role. But we need to look at the entire woman—her symptoms, her medical concerns, her mood, and her quality of life. This type of care involves a team of physicians, physician assistants, nurses, nurse practitioners, and mental health professionals. Exercise physiologists and nutritionists can also be extremely helpful. Also important are the CAM therapies—complementary and alternative medicine treatments such as acupuncture, chiropractic, and massage.

Accountability is another mutually important value. A physician, using evidence-based medicine, can help you make choices, but you must be an advocate and be able to participate in the decision. This type of partnership will provide the best health care.

Accountability also means being honest, even if that honesty is difficult. From the doctor's point of view, this may involve giving bad news. This may be a message like "The good news is that tamoxifen can reduce your risk of a breast cancer recurrence, but it will probably increase your hot flashes." The physician can then help a woman find other treatments for hot flashes, but the woman makes a decision based on knowledge.

As patients, we may have some difficulty being forthcoming as well. For example, we may not want to admit that we stopped taking a medication the doctor prescribed or began using an herbal product a friend recommended. We might downplay our sedentary habits or smoking or alcohol use or abuse of medications. Yet it is better to reveal the data. Most doctors will appreciate your honesty, and remember, you're not the first patient to tell them about unhealthy habits.

Cheryl gave all of these factors some thought. Over time she came to see that she had generally been treated with respect. Although her doctor had not relied on evidence-based medicine when she'd prescribed hormone therapy, her beliefs were quite consistent with those of other health care professionals, and fortunately she seemed to have escaped from harm. So Cheryl's anger dissipated. She decided to transfer her care but wrote her previous doctor a short note when she requested that her records be transferred.

When It's Not Necessarily Hormones

Veronica's situation was a bit different. She had implemented her plan, stopped taking her low-dose oral contraceptives, but didn't feel significantly better. She cried less often and felt more in control, though, so she was pleased with her decision. Still, her other symptoms of depression—lack of interest and concentration, sadness, and some suicidal thoughts—remained. It became clear that Veronica was suffering not from the blues or mood swings, but from a major depressive episode.

So she went to Plan B. Veronica decided to return to psychotherapy and take an antidepressant medication. It was wise for Veronica to take action. Once a person has had an episode of depression, there is a 50 percent chance for a recurrence, and up to 33 percent of depressive episodes can become a chronic form of depression. Sometimes this happens because the original episode of depression was not truly treated. If Veronica could eliminate her symptoms now, she would not only feel better but also perhaps avoid future episodes. She and her psychiatrist chose fluoxetine (Prozac), a medication that had helped Veronica in the past. The SSRIs, or selective serotonin reuptake inhibitors, increase the available amount of serotonin, a neurotransmitter that helps improve mood. In addition, a study found that fluoxetine helped reduce hot flashes. Although this was not a major factor for Veronica, it was an additional benefit.

In psychotherapy, Veronica realized that there were many positive things in her life: She enjoyed her work. She and Sybil had a peaceful and strong relationship. They had a network of friends and enjoyed hiking, listening to music, and going to the movies. Nevertheless, her father's declining health and deterioration from alcoholism cast a dark shadow over her present life. Even though her parents were financially secure and living in Arizona, Veronica came to realize that she was angry and sad about both her parents—her father for his substance abuse and her mother for never really confronting or leaving her father.

Veronica and her psychotherapist were working on several issues related to alcohol and depression. Veronica may well have inherited a predisposition to substance abuse and depression. Although she had worked hard to establish a happy and productive life, she still felt echoes of sadness and guilt. So Veronica and her therapist were considering helping her mother hospitalize her father in a unit specializing in geriatric psychiatry. Veronica wanted to give this a try but was realistic about the potential barriers. Her therapist and she worked with an alcohol intervention specialist in Arizona.

An added benefit of this discussion was that it led to Veronica's revealing that she and Sybil tended to drink a bottle of wine together most evenings. As was mentioned in Chapter 4, even drinking the equivalent of two drinks (two 5-ounce glasses of wine) per night put both women at risk for such alcohol-related problems as liver damage and an increased risk of breast cancer. Veronica, in addition, should not have been drinking much at all, since alcohol is a depressant. She decided to quit drinking, and Sybil, who was concerned about breast cancer, decided to cut back, too, limiting her intake to one glass of wine per night.

Unlike Terry's difficulties with sleep and moods, Veronica's depression was only tangentially related to her perimenopause. The low-dose contraceptive may have triggered or worsened her mood. Most women who become depressed between the ages of 45 and 55 are like Veronica, with high levels of family stress and/or a history of depression.

After twelve weeks on the fluoxetine, Veronica found that her mood had improved significantly. She no longer had any suicidal ideas and had much improved energy. She knew that she had to deal with her parents, but with the help of a psychotherapist, Sybil, and some close friends, she was ready to try.

Your Plan

Use your diaries in a similar fashion. Notice and try to eliminate any barriers to your plan. If you are taking medications, are you doing so consistently? If you are having any troubling side effects, check with your physician or pharmacist. You can find out whether they will decrease over time, or perhaps taking a medication at a different time of day will help. Perhaps a similar medication with fewer side effects can be prescribed.

If you are working on a lifestyle change, try to reward yourself periodically. If you are having difficulties maintaining your plan, do what we did with Cheryl and try to learn from any slips. Keep trying. Get support. Reevaluate. Try again.

Now look over your diary and pay attention to the symptoms. If there has been some change, excellent. If not, and if you have been implementing your plan consistently, then it's time to talk with your doctor. As in these cases, you can fine-tune your plan as needed. If you keep at it, your plan will work.

CHAPTER NINE

○─○─○

Creative Thoughts and Strong Bonds

Menopause is really just a biological marker—the end of menstruation. This turning point has a unique meaning for each woman. For some, it is a bittersweet reminder of the passage of time. Some women may have regrets about their fertility, about whether and when they had children. For still others, it is a marker of freedom—no more fears of unwanted pregnancy, no tampons, fewer responsibilities. In some cultures, menopause is the entrée to the male world of privilege and respect. But whatever menopause means to you, we want to help you deal with any medical symptoms you may have as well as the implications of them. Then we want you to move on and enjoy your life.

This chapter will help you develop your psychological strength and expand your social network. After all, no matter what medical issues you face, if you've developed some psychological resilience and a strong support system, you will feel stronger and be better able to cope.

What can go wrong during our midlife years? Unfortunately, a lot. Health issues may become more frequent and more complex. We may feel we have less stamina. Sometimes we suffer a loss—divorce or the death of a friend or family member. And because women still provide the lion's share of caretaking, the health and safety concerns for our family members multiply as we grow older, too.

But even when troubles add up, our coping skills are usually more mature and better developed in midlife than when we were younger. Some specific psychological strategies have been shown to promote health and well-being. One is to defeat the fear of aging. We have found that just beneath the surface of many midlife women is the fear that "I am old now," or worse: "This is the beginning of the end." Although this is a belief that is hard to escape in our youth-oriented culture, there are ways not to adopt it.

While there's nothing wrong with staying young-looking, we need to focus on health and activity rather than on surface appeal. The actor Debra Winger suggested that the best way to cope with growing older is to cut down on the number of mirrors in your home! After all, it is ultimately a losing battle if your goal is to look young forever. On the other hand, we can *act* and *think* forever young. When the actor Ruth Gordon was asked about being 80 years old, she replied, "I think of myself as *aging*, not *aged*. Everyone ages. Toddlers. Teenagers. It's a process."

Psychological science supports this view. A study by two psychologists at University of Pittsburgh, Joyce Bromberger and Karen Matthews, looked at an important question: What makes women vulnerable to depression at midlife? Depression continues to plague midlife women as it does women of all ages, although to a lesser degree than younger women, contrary to the popular stereotype. Drs. Bromberger and Matthews examined traits that are typically seen as being feminine to see if they put women at greater risk for a midlife depression.

Studying 460 women volunteers who were part of a larger study of women, menopause, and heart disease, they looked at the women's scores on the Beck Depression Inventory (a widely used questionnaire to measure depression) and life stress. In addition, they focused on four traits: One was the ability to express anger, as opposed to suppressing it. Another was something they called private self-consciousness—the degree to which the women attended to their private thoughts, feelings, and bodily sensations. They also looked at stressful life events and chronic difficulties, such as financial problems. Finally, they assessed whether women were instrumental—that is, focused on action—versus expressive, focusing on feelings.

The results were somewhat surprising. Many have suggested that women are depressed because they are sensitive and highly nurturing to others. These characteristics could lead to emotional depletion and depression. But Drs. Bromberger and Matthews did not find this to be true.

But three other traits did correlate with depression—being passive, suppressing anger, and a high degree of private self-consciousness. Women who are prone to mood problems tend to ruminate or brood. It's a type of morbid meditation. In general, women brood much more often than men, especially in response to mood. Although there are often good reasons for our brooding, we need to break the cycle. Otherwise, negativism or irritability can become a lifestyle.

Coping by Distraction: Why Can't a Woman Be More Like a Man?

As women, we have been taught to be the mood experts. From an early age, girls are encouraged both at home and at school to reflect on their feelings and to take responsibility for the feelings of others. This is a healthy socialization process that encourages self-awareness and a sense of connection. Taken to the extreme, however, it can lead to a lack of action or self-assertion and even clinical depression. When the necessary balance between action and reflection is lost, the brooding becomes a habit.

Men, on the other hand, are usually taught too much about behavior and rules. Boys are still told to suck it up and act like a man. Or they are encouraged to do something physical, to go outside and play. The positive result is that they become doers and can take charge. When faced with a mood problem, they can be experts at action and distraction. Yet taken to the extreme, the socialization process neglects the world of feelings and men can lose their emotional vocabularies.

Neither extreme is desirable. For men, it can lead to denial and repression of emotions, increased risk of heart disease, and the problems associated with dangerous distractions. Many experts believe that the high rate of alcohol and drug abuse in men reflects an inability to cope with sad feelings. In women, a habit of brooding may make us prone to clinical depression or the less serious but more constant states of moodiness, anxiety, or pessimism. Sad or irritable moods occur so often in women that we tend to view them as normal.

But what is the difference between healthy self-assessment and rumination or brooding? You know that you are brooding when:

- You find that you're thinking about only one issue for long periods of time.
- You are focusing on your responsibility alone, overlooking that of the other people involved.
- You are thinking in circles—going round and round without reaching new conclusions.
- When you approach the subject, you feel a sense of dread or hopelessness.
- You lose sleep over the problem because you are worrying.

What can we conclude from this and other studies? Erik Erickson described eight stages of life. Each stage had a polarity, or tension, between two psychological tasks. Erickson suggested that the midlife polarity is between generativity and self-absorption. So we can become overly self-focused and worry about thoughts, feelings, aches, and pains, or we can focus on productive worth and on contributing to the next generation. The joy and involvement of work of any kind can pull us away from midlife brooding. The work can be paid or volunteer, a traditional career or contribution to a family or friendship network. We have found that involvement and expression of values are two important elements. Many women at midlife are fortunate in that they now have more time and resources to work on causes that are significant to them—justice, equality, or environmental issues, to name a few.

Another option is just to have some fun. Yes, pure fun. Many women need to learn about distraction. When mired in a problem that seems hopeless, do something different. Leave the area. Create a list of distracting activities. Here's the start of a sample list:

- Watch Comedy Central on TV
- Listen to old Motown tunes

- Participate in a step aerobics class
- Drink tea while reading a mystery novel

And so on. You get the idea. Not easy if you are a brooder, but worth trying.

New Perspectives

Midlife can be the perfect time to explore new and old interests, careers, passions, and self-knowledge in general. It has long been understood that midlife brings an awareness of the finite nature of life. This leads naturally to reflection and self-expression. In addition, by midlife women may be less self-conscious than they were in their youth.

We've found that many women pick up strands of past interests; they might resume their education, for example, or take up singing or playing an instrument. There are community and university education programs all over the country that can spark and develop these pursuits.

As women who write, we also believe in the healing power of words. Writing and reading can help you through hard times. That is why so many women take up journal writing at midlife. It allows privacy and reflection and creativity. Reading also inspires us. So many women have passed before us. We can take comfort and gain power from their words. Anne Tyler's novel *Back When We Were Grown-ups*, for example, helps us understand the midlife transition. When the book opens, Rebecca, a 53-year-old widow, faces multigenerational family responsibilities, yet she feels that she has lost herself: "Once upon a time there was a woman who discovered she had turned into the wrong person."

Rebecca rediscovers her college boyfriend, Will, who is now divorced, and sees him for a few months. Over time she sees that they are not a good match. Throughout this process she reevaluates her life. Ultimately she embraces her role in the extended family and comes to value what she does well: "Now she saw that her most valuable contribution had been her joyousness. . . . Not that she per se was joyous to begin with. No. She had had to tutor it. . . . Finally she experimented with a sneaking sense of achievement. Pride, even."

Rebecca eventually recognizes her immense contribution to four generations of her extended family. Other women discover additional avenues for generosity through mentoring younger colleagues or volunteering in their community or becoming politically active. Like Rebecca, they realize that there are many dreams left to be explored: "There were still so many happenings yet to be hoped for in her life."

Social Support: What Women Do Best

But perhaps the most powerful midlife tool is social connection and support. Intimacy can help us through the worst of times. Take a moment. Sit back and try to remember the last time you felt one of the following emotions: Perhaps you felt understood—that another person was able to listen to you and actually felt how you felt. Or perhaps you felt a sense of kinship—that is, you shared something in common. It could be something wonderful like the birth of a new child or something tragic such as an illness in the family. Or when did you last just share a good laugh with someone? Perhaps you were at the movies, watching television, or just talking. All of these three experiences— empathy, similarity, and humor—are aspects of intimacy.

We can think of social support as an individual, family, or group phenomenon. Drs. Brown and Harris provided a classic example of individual social support in a landmark study of women at risk to become depressed. In their book *Social Origins of Depression* (1978), they describe poor, uneducated single mothers in a London neighborhood who were under enormous stress, financially and otherwise. The study found that having a close confidant—someone to talk to and share problems with—was a buffer to clinical depression.

Many later studies have found consistent results. For example, in a more recent project from the Boston College School of Social Work, the authors looked at the influence of social relationship factors on women's adjustment to cancer. The forty-nine women in this study were receiving treatments such as chemotherapy or radiation for cancer, had at least one child age 12 and younger, and had received their cancer diagnosis between two and thirty-six months before the beginning of the study. The authors looked at the patients' quality of life, depression, ability to take care of themselves, and mutuality of close relationships. The self-silencing scale created by Dana Crowley Jack was used to understand how much women felt they could speak up, and the extent to which they sacrificed for the needs of others. With respect to relationships, the researchers looked at two parts. Engagement was the extent to which a partner would be involved with the patient and coping with the illness, whereas protective buffering occurred when a partner is excluded to avoid disagreement or to protect him from the disturbing situation.

The results of this study confirmed the importance of social support. The women who had mutuality in their relationships and fewer self-silencing beliefs had a more positive psychosocial adaptation to cancer. Perceiving their partner relationships to be highly mutual was a significant positive predictor of the patients' high quality of life, lack of depression, and ability to take care of themselves.

The study looked not only at what a woman *received* from her partner but at what she *gave* as well. When a woman has a serious illness it is important for her to continue to feel that she is fully participating and supporting her partner as well as receiving support. It was this mutuality, or shared sense of relationship, that also empowered these women to feel better able to take care of themselves.

In contrast, the silencing of the self was seen as detrimental during this time of coping with serious illness. Although self-silencing was found not to be related to either depression or psychological well-being, it was found to affect the woman's ability to take care of herself. The women who attempted to protect or buffer their family members from the stress of their illness did not cope well. The burden was just too great.

Also noteworthy, although this was a small group of woman, was that such illness-related issues as symptoms, length of sickness, and socioeconomic status did not affect a woman's psychosocial adaptation. So it shows us another good example of the power of connection.

Social cohesiveness looks at the extent to which a group of people, neighborhood, or family sticks together. Two of the most important qualities are trust and dependability. Ask yourself, "Whom could I call in the middle of the night without worrying that I would bother them?" For some women, their families of origin may not be the most supportive. Even then, they can establish new families, which may be composed of neighbors, close friends, or coworkers who have common bonds and a commitment to care for each other.

Social support is important, but so is just plain socializing. Virtually anything that puts us in contact with other people—having a spouse or partner, face-to-face interactions with good friends, or keeping in touch long distance and even by e-mail—improves our quality of life. Scholars at the Harvard School of Public Health followed 2,800 men and women who were older than 65. Over a twelve-year period, they asked two sets of questions. One was a group of questions about ten general and personal changes, and the other was designed to look at cognitive changes. The research also looked at social engagement. The conclusion was that a decline in social activity increased the risk of cognitive decline and even early death. While this could occur because people tend to withdraw from social activities when they become ill, those who showed a loss in cognitive function were those who were more likely to score low on their social interaction test from the outset. So social support can keep our minds alert and improve our health.

Another interesting study from Penn State University looked at the psychological benefits derived from receiving holiday cards. They found that adults from the age of 24 to 87 all liked to get cards, but for different reasons. Younger people found that the cards were a way to build or maintain their social connections, whereas older people viewed the cards as a link to their past. In both sets of people, half the cards were from respondents that the people hadn't seen for more than a year. The more cards people received, the more connected they felt.

It is also important to look at what social support is *not*. The pure number of friends does not equal the degree of social support. Quality is more important than the quantity of time, although we should not delude ourselves into thinking that the quantity of time can be reduced to practically nothing. Reciprocity is important or friendship can be draining.

Working patterns and gender roles have affected social support in another surprising way. When women went to work outside the home, we brought with us many of our expectations about relationships: that they would be caring, that they would be social, that there would be rituals at work—birthday parties, baby showers, and so on. Those of you who are working outside the home might look around the office and notice who provides these events and these connections. It's usually the women. On the one hand, our social needs are probably improving the workplace. On the other hand, we are also increasing our number of responsibilities at work without decreasing them at home. So a positive aspect is that you may have social connections at work, but there's a danger of becoming emotionally depleted if you don't have help and support.

Five Steps to Midlife Social Support

1. Recognize that social support is important not only to your psychological but also to your physical health. Many women will see the need for social support when we point out that it might lengthen their life or help them cope with illness, but it also has the power to improve our overall sense of well-being.

2. Do an assessment. Who can you count on? Not just to call in the middle of the night: Who would help out with your family or your kids if you needed it? With whom can you share your job problems? Who really listens to you when you have a problem at home?

3. Take *action*. Looking at the list of supports, you might find it lacking or might realize that there was someone who was once close to you but is no longer. Scan your emotional horizons. There may well be someone in your social network with the potential to become a friend. Understand that people change over time. There may be a sibling, friend, or cousin with whom you always felt fairly close, but something impeded intimacy. Perhaps you became alienated from one another, or perhaps the environment wasn't right. Look again. Take time to reevaluate and build on those relationships.

   Do you have acquaintances whom you sense could become better friends? If you feel there's potential for mutuality or connection, follow up. One way to decide whether you can get social support from a friend is to evaluate whether you feel better or worse after seeing her or him. If you always feel exhausted afterward, then perhaps you're in one of those relationships that is not mutual.

   Maybe you don't have the feeling of intimacy and intense communication, but you have a good buddy. You have a good time together, share similar senses of humor, or have common interests. That's helpful, too. One person doesn't have to fill all your needs. Value the importance of social support, scan

your emotional horizons, try to build on old relationships or
rekindle them, or develop new ones.

4. Join self-help groups or community institutions. Tradition-
ally, religious and educational institutions have been the
foundations of support for families. Volunteer work through
hospitals and community agencies can also provide this feeling of support and of contribution—which is another way to
feel the sense of connection. By helping someone else, you
can learn more about yourself.

In 1993 there were more than 15 million people in the
United States who attended 500,000 different self-help groups
every week, and that number has grown. The social support
provided by self-help groups can expand our social network.
And if you think back to three of the experiences described
earlier—a sense of empathy, similarity, and humor—you can
see that all of these can exist in self-help groups, along with a
fair amount of practical support.

5. The time is now. Midlife is often a series of existential
moments. It is after all the time when the question "How
much time do I have left?" becomes more real. So now is
the time to change your life. Or to enhance it. Or to appreciate it.

Although midlife can be challenging, it also brings new opportunities. We are usually wiser, less easily embarrassed, less preoccupied with
making people like us. After all, if we become invisible, then we might
as well be able to do what we want! Who is watching?

We can also work against female stereotypes by expressing our
feelings, including that taboo feeling of anger, more directly. We can
defeat brooding by staying actively involved in life. We can cherish our
relationships, grow, and move on. In the final chapter we will help you
use all sorts of resources to continue your education in women's health.

CHAPTER TEN

○—○—○

Expanding Your
Knowledge

We hope you've gained confidence in your ability to make decisions about menopause, and we also hope that you feel our support and the support of the other women who have successfully navigated this midlife transition.

But how will you continue to expand your knowledge about menopause and women's health? The past few years have been extremely confusing for any woman who wants to make decisions based on women's health research. Many of the assumptions of the medical profession have been proven to be wrong. Even the experts seem to be a bit perplexed. Many women are anxious and uncertain. Still, new research is needed to clarify the many unanswered questions. Fortunately, though, there are more excellent resources available to you than ever. Remember, no one has all the new information, so keep your ears and eyes open.

This brings us to our philosophy of using government resources. You want your information to be research-based, well written, and preferably free! Hence, federal government resources are a good bet. They are extensive and often refer you to additional organizations. When in doubt, start at the National Women's Health Information Center at www.4women.org. It is a referral service offered by the Department of Health and Human Services. The phone number is 1-800-994-WOMAN (1-800-994-9662) or 1-888-220-5446 for the hearing impaired. The information referral specialists there speak both English and Spanish. The office is open from 9:00 A.M. until 6:00 P.M. EST. Why not benefit from our tax dollars at work? This is the most efficient way to access reliable information.

When you are exploring the recommended resources, pay attention to your learning style. Which type of media is most helpful to you? Print, CD-ROMs, lectures? If you've gotten this far in the book, then obviously the written word is appealing to you. So you might benefit from reading other books or subscribing to a women's health newsletter. The *Harvard Women's Health Watch*, available in print or online at http://www.health.harvard.edu/. There are also pamphlets available from nonprofit associations. We have included a section detailing the books, magazines, and brochures available.

For those of you who like to watch television or listen to the radio, there are a few options. With the demise of Lifetime Medical Television, the only national channel that addresses medical concerns is the Discovery Channel. They have periodic shows on women's health. Your local Public Broadcasting System (PBS) channel may have a program from time to time, as does National Public Radio (NPR). If you are a television watcher, though, beware of infomercials! We haven't seen any specifically on menopause yet, but it is only a matter of time. Numerous unsubstantiated health claims are made for the variety of products advertised. They may appear to be documentaries or evidence-based, but they are actually very long commercials aimed at selling a product.

We enjoy interactive learning seminars because we can discover what other women are thinking. Workshops or lectures and panels offer a lot of give-and-take. Many university adult education divisions, hospitals, and medical schools offer these.

The Internet and Other Sources: All Information, All the Time, and Lots of It Wrong

The Internet has transformed our lives. Never before has the average person had access to so much medical information. You are one click away from the National Library of Medicine, medical and psychological journals, self-help groups, and international experts in women's health. That's the good news. The bad news is that you are also one click away from savvy quacks, charlatans, and entrepreneurs. Anyone with a bit of training can create a Web site, fraudulently put the title Dr. in front of his or her name, and start giving advice. Unlike professional journals, there is no peer review. Many Web sites are merely marketing tools for products without any scientific basis to their claims.

So the most attractive Web sites may not be the most reputable; they are merely the most graphically stimulating. On the other hand, some Web sites are professionally operated and include sound advice, but are supported by pharmaceutical companies. This is reasonable, but you should notice sponsor organizations. This clues you in to the site's particular point of view and potential biases.

How can you use the Internet as one of the tools to help guide you through menopause without being overwhelmed or exploited? Don't just put the term *menopause* into a search engine. If you do, you will get over 1 million links. The first few are the sponsored sites, often profit-making sites designed as sales tools for various remedies. Here's a better plan. It is always worthwhile to check with your primary care professional to see if he or she has a favorite reliable Web site. Then you will be on the same page (or site) as him or her and will be able to discuss current findings. If not, you can start at www.4women.org for information related to women's health.

If you want another review of the status of hormone therapy, there is a wonderful and extensive site titled Facts About Postmenopausal Hormone Therapy at http://www.nhlbi.nih.gov/health/women/pht_facts.htm. This site brings you up-to-date results from the Women's Health Initiative and lists the various formulations of hormones.

If you want information about complementary and alternative medicine (CAM) or herbal remedies, remember that the research in this area is relatively new. Also, as previously discussed, there are fewer safeguards for herbal remedies: With a prescription medication the industry has to prove that a medication is safe before it is released to the public. With an herbal supplement, the situation is reversed; a supplement can be released and the consumer or the government has to prove that it is unsafe. Again, www.4women.org will provide links to the appropriate sites. Or you can go directly to www.nccam.nih.gov. Here you will discover extensive information about CAM from the National Institutes of Health. The site includes health alerts and a list of ongoing clinical trials. Another good resource for CAM is www.herbalgram.org, a site that reviews herbal remedies and is sponsored by the nonprofit research-based America Botanical Council. It also presents data on side effects and interactions with medications.

If you have questions about either prescribed or over-the-counter (OTC) medications, you should consult with your health care professional or a pharmacist. The FDA maintains a Web site for women, www.fda.gov/womens/default.htm. Here you can follow the estrogen and progestin controversy, as the site includes news releases, labeling changes, and new research. In addition, you can sign up for the FDA's Consumer Digest, a magazine available online or in print. You can also log on to www.CVS.com, an online pharmacy that provides specific information about medications as well as articles about health.

The Internet, though, is not the safest place to purchase remedies. If you read about something that seems too good to be true, it probably is. ("Cheap! Effective! Special Offer for New Customers!") Remember the placebo effect. Remember that many remedies are unregulated. Some Web sites promote specific medications, without helping you evaluate your symptoms or the medication within your overall health care. Not a good idea.

Other important aspects of midlife health are prevention, nutrition, and exercise. The *Tufts University Health and Nutrition Letter* at http://healthletter.tufts.edu includes sections on all these topics. It allows you to sample free articles before subscribing. An emphasis on strength training is one of the most exciting changes in health maintenance for midlife women. The best books are in the *Strong Women Stay*

Young (Stay Smart, Stay Slim, and so forth) series. The series is coauthored by Miriam Nelson, Ph.D., a director of the Center for Physical Activities and Nutrition at Tufts University. The Web site is www.strongwomen.com and is based on solid clinical research.

Finally, don't forget the psychological aspect of your health! The National Institute of Mental Health, www.nimh.nih.gov, has a section for the public with information about depression and anxiety. It has an extensive publication list for other conditions as well. So do the American Psychological Association, www.apa.org, and the American Psychiatric Association, www.psychiatry.org. The American Association of Marriage and Family Therapists offers articles about family problems and developmental issues at www.aamft.org/families/index_nm.asp. All of these professional organizations also provide a therapist referral network, as does the National Association of Social Workers at www.socialworkers.org. The National Coalition Against Domestic Violence, www.ncadv.org, provides information, support, and phone numbers of hotlines and agencies.

We've given you many of the best national Web sites, but many local medical schools and hospitals also include patient education information on their Web sites. So you can do a search on menopause within, for example, "Springfield Medical School." You'll discover research-based information, along with notices about clinical or research programs or support groups.

Once you've done your research, you can return to your health care professional with new ideas or suggestions. When discussing your findings, it's best to cite the specific source rather than say, "I read about this on the Internet." (Remember, you can read about anything on the Internet.) Rather, you can say, "I read this on the NIH Web site" or "Springfield Medical Center is evaluating this treatment," or better still, print the information and take it with you to the appointment. If the material is new to your physician, she or he will then be able to find the precise Web site and area of concern.

If you don't have a computer or you're not adept at using the Internet, ask a librarian. Most local libraries have Internet access as well as helpful reference librarians. Or you can call and ask for information; in Resources we have included phone numbers as well as Web site information for many major organizations.

The Internet is just one of many ways to keep up-to-date. Use it in conjunction with your other resources, including print media, materials from your primary care physician, and most of all, the knowledge you've gained and your own common sense to help you stay current about menopause and your other health concerns.

Some Final Thoughts

Sometimes the words *menopausal* or *postmenopausal* are used to describe all that there is to know about midlife women. Yet it is important not to allow ourselves to be characterized in this fashion nor to internalize these labels. Why? Because to accept them is to reduce women to their reproductive status. We know that any individual woman is more than the sum of her hormone levels. Certainly hormones do play a role in midlife health. We've covered the health implications of menopause as well as the decisions that need to be considered. But we need to remember the big picture. The big picture is the answer to the question: How can we live long, healthy, active, and happy lives?

Some of the books in the Resources are stories of the lives of midlife women. They reveal that we are so much more than hormones or the lack thereof. Menopause can be an existential time, a time for us to appreciate every day. The Academy Award–winning film *The Hours* was based on the novel by the same name by Michael Cunningham. The film is moving and well crafted, but as is often the case, loses some of the book's beautiful words. Knowing that life brings much sadness and at times serious illness, Cunningham writes:

> There's just this for consolation: an hour here or there when our lives seem, against all odds and expectations, to burst open and give us everything we've ever imagined, though everyone but children (and perhaps even they) knows these hours will inevitably be followed by others, far darker and more difficult. Still we cherish the city, the morning; we hope, more than anything, for more.

Take good care of yourself and enjoy what the rest of your life has to offer.

Resources

Web Sites

American Cancer Society
www.cancer.org
The ACS is a national voluntary health organization committed to education and research in the fight against cancer. The site provides a general overview, a detailed guide, links to more information, and an interactive treatment decision tool for help with choices regarding your own care. It is also a resource for support and community organizations.

American Heart Association
www.americanheart.org
Heart disease and stroke affect one out of two women and can be prevented. This Web site presents a wealth of information about cardiovascular disease including risk factors, signs and symptoms, preventable lifestyle tips, treatment options, and the latest research findings.

Food and Drug Administration–Office of Women's Health
www.fda.gov/womens
The FDA has jurisdiction over the drugs, medical devices, vaccines, blood and tissue products, foods, and cosmetics approved for use by American consumers. This Web site is a resource for prevention and treatments recommended to women based on the research used by the FDA to make its determinations.

National Cancer Institute
www.cancer.org
This site provides cancer information from the National Cancer Institute. It includes cancer information, clinical trials, statistics, and research programs. A special feature is PDQ (Physician Data Query), which is a NCI database of latest information about cancer treatment, screening, prevention, clinical trials, genetics, and supportive care.

National Breast Cancer Foundation
www.thebreastcancersite.com
One Hanover Park
16633 North Dallas Parkway, Suite 600
Addison, TX 75001
206-268-5400
This organization offers information and news updates about the early detection and treatment of breast cancer. The site has corporate sponsors. You can go to "Click here" at the site and help fund free mammograms for women who need them. According to their reports, 20 percent of the funds raised are for administration, while 80 percent go directly for funding the mammograms.

National Coalition Against Domestic Violence
www.ncadv.org
NCADV is dedicated to the elimination of personal and societal violence. The Web site provides information on abusive relationships and steps women can take to prevent and end battering in their lives. Hotlines to call and links to local agencies to contact for help are included.

National Institute of Mental Health
www.nimh.nih.gov
The NIMH is devoted to the achievement of better understanding, treatment, and prevention of mental illness. The section of this Web site entitled *For the Public* offers information about the most common disorders, including those affecting women, including depression, anxiety disorders, and eating disorders.

National Osteoporosis Foundation–Prevention of Osteoporosis
www.nof.org/prevention/index.htm
Osteoporosis-related information helps viewers find doctors in their area and presents news and events as well as research information on osteoporosis prevention. Updates and historical information help viewers understand prevention, treatment, and education.

North American Menopause Society
www.menopause.org
The North American Menopause Society is one of the largest and oldest professional organizations devoted to menopause. They have excellent materials for consumers available as well as links to dozens of other sites that are considered worthwhile by the society. NAMS also publishes Menopause Flashes, a free monthly e-mail newsletter for

consumers, with information about menopause, perimenopause, early menopause, and the many therapies available.

U.S. Preventative Services Task Force
www.ahrq.gov/clinic/prevnew.htm
The U.S. Preventative Services Task Force offers *The Guide to Clinical Preventative Services*, which provides the latest available recommendations on preventative interventions, including screening tests, counseling, and immunizations for more than 80 conditions. It is updated regularly.

Newsletters and Magazines

A Friend Indeed
Main Floor—419 Graham Avenue
Winnipeg, MB R3C 0M3 Canada
Or
Box 260
Pembina, ND 58271
204-989-8028
204-898-8028
www.afriendindeed.ca
This grandmother of all menopause newsletters was founded by Janine O'Leary Cobb and is now published by the Women's Health Clinic of Winnipeg. Each issue includes a feature article as well as new research. An annual subscription for six issues costs $30.

Dr. Andrew Weil's Self-Healing: Creating Natural Health for Your Body and Mind
Thorne Communications, Inc.
42 Pleasant Street
Watertown, MA 02472
Toll free U.S./Canada: 800-523-3296
www.drweilselfhealing.com
Dr. Andrew Weil publishes this monthly alternative medicine newsletter. An annual subscription of twelve issues costs $18 (U.S.).

Harvard Women's Health Watch
PO Box 420068
Palm Coast, FL 32142
Toll free U.S./Canada: 800-829-5921

Outside U.S./Canada: 904-445-4662
www.health.harvard.edu/
Edited by faculty from Harvard Medical School, this newsletter
addresses a wide range of health issues. The annual subscription of
twelve issues costs $32 for U.S. subscribers or $40 (U.S.) for Canadian
subscribers.

HerbalGram

American Botanical Council
PO Box 144345
Austin, TX 78714
Toll free U.S./Canada: 800-373-7105
Outside U.S./Canada: 512-331-8868
www.herbalgram.org
The American Botanical Council and Herb Research Foundation
jointly publish this newsletter. It has an editorial board of leading scientists in the field of herbal pharmacology. It details the use of herbs
for a variety of health effects and provides a comprehensive list of
resources. A subscription of four issues is free with an annual member-
ship fee of $50; outside the U.S. add $20 (U.S.).

Living Beyond Breast Cancer

www.lbbc.org or call the Survivors' Helpline at 888-753-5222
This quarterly educational newsletter covers many aspects of life after
a breast cancer diagnosis. It is free.

Stress Control: Techniques for Preventing and Easing Stress

Special Health Report, Harvard Medical School
Harvard Health Publications
PO Box 421073
Palm Coast, FL 32142-1073
www.health.harvard.edu/reports
Stress control experts Herbert Benson, M.D., and Alice Domar, Ph.D.,
developed this report. It helps readers identify situations that trigger
stress and also spells out the many ways stress can impact negatively on
health. Copies are $16 each.

The Newsletter of Nutrition, Fitness, and Self-Care

University of California, School of Public Health, Berkeley Wellness
Letter
www.WellnessLetter.com

This newsletter focuses on both prevention and health in general, presenting health-driven facts and steps to using them. Nutrition and exercise are specific areas of expertise.

Tufts University Health & Nutrition Letter: Your Guide to Living Healthier Longer
Tufts University
PO Box 420235
Palm Coast, FL 32142
Toll free U.S./Canada: 800-274-7581
Outside U.S./Canada: 617-350-7994
www.healthletter.tufts.edu
This newsletter, published by one of the leading nutrition research centers in the United States, offers current, scientific advice about diet and its effects on health. Some articles also address other lifestyle issues. The cost for an annual subscription of twelve issues is $28; the newsletter is also available on the Web site.

Booklets

U.S. Public Health Service
You Can Quit Smoking. Consumer Booklet, September 2002. Available at http://www.surgeongeneral.gov/tobacco/lowlit/htm.

Boning Up on Osteoporosis: A Guide to Prevention and Treatment
National Osteoporosis Foundation
P.O. Box 930299
Atlanta, GA 31193-0299
Toll free U.S./Canada: 877-868-4520
Outside U.S./Canada: 202-223-2226
This is a 70-page booklet that was updated in 1998 and costs $3. Individual copies of a smaller booklet, *Menopause and Osteoporosis*, are available for $0.45. You may also join the organization for $15 a year and receive both booklets free as well as other membership benefits.

MenoPak Program
North American Menopause Society
PO Box 94527
Cleveland, OH 44101

440-442-7550
NAMS offers the widest range of well-written educational materials for consumers and professionals. The MenoPak costs $5 and includes a menopause guidebook and reading list.

Menopause: Let's Talk About It, 2000 edition
The Osteoporosis Society of Canada
Toronto, Ontario
Toll free: 800-463-6842
The Osteoporosis Society of Canada and the Society of Obstetricians and Gynaecologists of Canada (two nonprofit organizations) produced this free booklet for Canadian women, but it is appropriate for all women. They can also provide fact sheets on the role of calcium, exercise, and hormone therapy.

Osteoporosis and You, 2001 edition
The Osteoporosis Society of Canada
Toronto, Ontario
Toll free: 800-463-6842
This free booklet is a good resource for any woman who wants an overview of osteoporosis and how to prevent it.

Understanding and Controlling Cholesterol, 2001 edition
American Heart Association
Dallas, TX
Toll free: 800-242-8721
Information about cholesterol and healthy eating is offered in this 28-page booklet. Consumers may request up to 10 brochures free of charge.

Understanding and Controlling Your High Blood Pressure, 2001 edition
American Heart Association
Dallas, TX
Toll free: 800-242-8721.
The various medication options are outlined in this simple straightforward 24-page booklet. Consumers may request up to 10 brochures free of charge.

Understanding Hysterectomy, 1999 edition
The American College of Obstetricians and Gynecologists
Washington, DC

202-484-3321
Basic facts and information about hysterectomy are reviewed. A single copy of this booklet is available free to consumers who send a self-addressed stamped envelope to the ACOG Resource Center, 409 12th Street, SW, PO Box 96920, Washington, DC 20090.

Wellness Made Easy: 365 Tips for Better Health
PO Box 420148
Palm Coast, FL 32142
386-447-6328
Editorial Board, University of California, Berkeley. Health Letter Associates, 1999. Self-explanatory and clever advice.

Women and Sleep, 2001 edition
National Sleep Foundation
Washington, DC
Toll free: 800-673-7533.
This free booklet addresses sleep issues specific to women, including sleep changes associated with menopause.

Books

General Women's Health

All About Eve: The Complete Guide to Women's Health and Well-Being. T. C. Semler. New York: HarperCollins, 1995. This easy-to-understand and comprehensive volume is based on interviews with over 300 experts in women's health.

Eat, Drink, and Be Healthy. W. C. Willett. New York: Simon & Schuster Source, 2001. This book provides extensive evidence of the links between proper nutrition and better health. Healthy recipes are included, and the text is well written and well researched, identifying a total diet that helps create a healthy lifestyle.

The Harvard Guide to Women's Health, 2nd ed. K. J. Carlson, S. A. Eisenstadt, and T. Ziporyn. Cambridge, Mass.: Harvard University Press, 1996. The two senior authors organize an annual course on women's health. The book makes their knowledge about the comprehensive approach to women's health accessible to the reader.

The Healthy Boomer: A No-Nonsense Midlife Health Guide for Women and Men. P. Edwards, M. Lhotsky, and T. Turner. Toronto, Ont.: McClelland & Steward, 1999. This straightforward book includes accurate information and good advice for both women and men dealing with midlife. It is engaging and optimistic.

Our Bodies, Ourselves for the New Century: A Book by and for Women. The Boston Women's Health Book Collective. New York: Touchstone, 1998. This grandmother of all women's health guides is part of a classic series. Its latest revision maintains the strong feminist perspective and continues to increase awareness of the need for information and choices. Sisterhood is still powerful.

Prime Time: The African American Woman's Complete Guide to Midlife Health and Wellness. M. H. Gaston, G. K. Porter, and J. E. Jones. New York: Ballantine Books, 2001. A physician and a psychologist wrote this extensive guide to midlife health and wellness. It includes self-care and coping strategies for midlife. It combines a practical attitude with many women's stories.

Strong Women Stay Young. M. E. Nelson and S. Wernick. New York: Bantam Books, 1997. One of the best books we've read in years. Tufts University's Miriam Nelson emphasizes the many benefits of strength training for women of all ages. The book provides programs for at home use or for the gym.

Women's Health and Wellness from Health Magazine. Birmingham Ala.: Oxmoor House, 2003. A good summary of the latest ideas and tips about women's health.

Diabetes

American Diabetes Association's Complete Guide to Diabetes, 3rd ed. Alexandria, Va.: American Diabetes Association, 2002. Large, detailed, comprehensive book, this is a must for those with diabetes.

Healthy Cookbooks

American Heart Association Low-Fat, Low-Cholesterol Cookbook: Heart-Healthy, Easy-to-Make Recipes That Taste Great, 2nd ed. American Heart Association. New York: Times Books, 1997.

The Healthy Kitchen: Recipes for a Better Body, Life and Spirit.
A. Weil and R. Daley. New York: Alfred A. Knopf, 2002.

Low-Fat Lies: High Fat Frauds and the Healthiest Diet in the World. K. Vigilante and M. Flynn. New York: Regnery Publishing, 1999.

Moosewood Restaurant New Classics: 350 Recipes for Homestyle Fun and Everyday Feasts. New York: Clarkson Potter Publishing, 2001.

1001 Lowfat Soups and Stews: From Elegant Classics to Hearty One-Pot Meals. Edited by Sue Spitzer with Linda R. Yoakam, R.D., M.S. Chicago: Surrey Books, 2002.

Heart Health

The Female Heart: The Truth About Women and Heart Disease.
M. J. Legato and C. Colman. New York: Quill Publishing, 2000.
Written by a professor of clinical medicine at Columbia College of Physicians and Surgeons, this book gives you the true story about the dangers of heart disease, as well as strategies to prevent it.

Outsmarting the Midlife Fat Cell: Winning Weight-Control Strategies for Women over 35 to Stay Fit Through Menopause. D. Waterhouse. New York: Hyperion, 1998. Most women struggle with their weight at midlife. This book reflects a good attitude and details a variety of weight control plans for women over 35.

Hysterectomy, Breast Cancer, and Induced Menopause

The Breast Cancer Notebook: The Healing Power of Reflection.
A. L. Stanton and G. Reed. Washington, D.C.: American Psychological Association, 2003. A tool for helping women cope with all aspects of breast cancer and its treatment.

Guide to Quality Breast Cancer Care. Available from the National Breast Cancer Coalition Fund (NBCCF), www.stopbreastcancer.org or 800-622-2838. This is an excellent reference, with lots of new vocabulary, decision-making strategies, and tips for communicating with health care professionals. It also includes information about how clinical trials work. Its philosophy can be empowering to all health consumers.

Hysterectomy: Before and After: A Comprehensive Guide to Preventing Preparing for and Maximizing Health After Hysterectomy. W. B. Cutler. New York: HarperCollins,1990. This book is a bit old but is a good reference if you are going to have a hysterectomy. It gives you a detailed sense of what to expect.

You Don't Need a Hysterectomy, 2nd ed. I. K. Strausz, M.D. New York: Perseus Publishing, 2001. Thus book, written by a gynecologist, offers alternatives to hysterectomy, especially for women with fibroids or chronic pain.

Memory

Improving Memory: Understanding and Preventing Age-Related Memory Loss, 2000 edition.
Harvard Health Publications
1100 Summer Street, 2nd Floor
Stamford, CT 06905
Toll free U.S./Canada: 877-649-9457
This is a special health report by the Harvard Medical School; it explores the causes of memory problems, available treatments, and tips for improving and maintaining memory as well.

Osteoporosis

Stand Tall! Every Woman's Guide to Preventing and Treating Osteoporosis. M. Notelovitz, D. Tonnessen, and S. Meeks. Florida: Triad Publishing Company, 1998. The first author is a gynecologist and expert on menopause. This book provides a good explanation of osteoporosis and covers nutrition, exercise, and medication management.

Strong Women, Strong Bones: Everything You Need to Know to Prevent, Treat, and Beat Osteoporosis. M. E. Nelson and S. Wernick. New York: Putnam, 2000. In another book written by Tufts University's Miriam Nelson, the exercise physiologist creates a program to keep women's bones healthy.

Psychological Issues and Behavioral Medicine

The Dance of Connection: How to Talk to Someone When You're Mad, Hurt, Scared, Frustrated, Insulted, Betrayed, or Desperate. H. Lerner. New York: HarperCollins, 2001.The latest from the psychologist and author of the Dance of Anger series. Practical advice with women's stories included to help you speak up.

Feeling Good: The New Therapy. D. D. Burns, New York: Avon Books, 1999. This is the best book about cognitive therapy for depression. It has numerous questionnaires and exercises that help you understand how negative thoughts can lead to depressed mood.

The Healing Connection: How Women Form Relationships in Therapy and in Life. J. B. Miller and I. P. Stiver. Boston: Beacon Press, 1992. Two leading scholars and psychotherapists describe the power of connection to help women grow.

Healing and the Mind. B. Moyers. New York: Bantam Doubleday Dell, 1993. This book is based on the PBS television series by the same name. Bill Moyers covers acupuncture, traditional Chinese medicine, and stress management programs in this engaging book. Also available from PBS on video.

Minding the Body, Mending the Mind. J. Borysenko. New York: Bantam Doubleday Dell, 1993. Dr. Borysenko is the cofounder and former director of the Mind/Body Clinic at Boston's Deaconess Hospital. The book covers deep relaxation to promote physical healing and stress management. (Also available on audiocassette.)

The Shelter of Each Other: Rebuilding Our Families. M. Pipher. New York: Putnam, 1996. The author of *Reviving Ophelia* helps us understand the need for supporting strong families. It includes many suggestions for individual and social change.

Say Goodnight to Insomnia. G. D. Jacobs. New York: Holt, 1999. The director of the Behavioral Medicine Insomnia Program at a Boston medical center describes therapy that combines relaxation and other techniques to treat sleep disorders. Although it is not directed exclusively to menopausal women, it is a good reference for those who want to learn more about sleep problems.

Trauma and Recovery. J. Herman. New York: Basic Books, 1997. Psychiatrist Judith Herman writes beautifully about the effects of trauma on the individual. She also compares sexual and physical abuse to war trauma and terrorism, putting them into an important context.

The Women's Concise Guide to Emotional Well-Being. K. J. Carlson, S. A. Eisenstadt, and T. Ziporyn. Cambridge, Mass.: Harvard University Press, 1997. The Harvard Primary Care of Women team provides solid information about mental health.

Women Who Worry Too Much: How to Break Free of Overthinking and Reclaim Your Life. S. Nolen-Hoeksema. New York: Holt, 2003. A noted psychology professor helps women stop overanalyzing and thus avoid depression.

Sexuality

For Women Only: A Revolutionary Guide to Overcoming Sexual Dysfunction and Reclaiming Your Sex Life. J. Berman, L. Berman, and E. Bunmiller. New York: Holt, 2001. Written by sisters, a urologist and psychotherapist, this book presents up-to-date research and a discussion of female sexual issues. They present the viewpoint that sexual problems usually have multiple causes.

For Yourself: The Fulfillment of Female Sexuality. L. Barbach. New York: Signet, 2000. Well-known for her work in this area, psychologist Lonnie Barbach provides a guide to female sexual functioning that is informative and practical.

History, Humor, and Inspiration

Back When We Were Grownups. Anne Tyler. New York: Ballantine Books, 2002. As always, Anne Tyler describes the struggles and joys of families better than just about anyone. In this novel, she explores the life and regrets of a midlife woman.

Menopause: The Silent Meow. M. Sacks. Berkeley, Calif.: Ten Speed Press, 1995. This one makes us laugh. This is a cute book of cat cartoons with humorous "hints" for dealing with menopausal problems. For example, both loss of sexual interest and too much sexual interest are solved by having affairs with younger cats.

On Women Turning 50: Celebrating Midlife Discoveries. C. Rountree. New York: HarperCollins, 1993. This is an optimistic anthology of interviews and photographs of such well-known women as Barbara Boxer and Cokie Roberts. Through prose and poems, they share their discoveries and feelings about growing older.

New and Selected Poems by Mary Oliver. Mary Oliver. Boston: Beacon Press, 1993. This volume won the National Book Award for poetry in 1992. The poems create a sense of serenity. Many of them describe the wonders of nature.

Poems of Audre Lorde. Audre Lorde. New York: W.W. Norton & Company, 2000. Audre Lorde was a brilliant African American lesbian poet who died of cancer too soon in 1992.

Wild Women in the Kitchen: 101 Rambunctious Recipes and 99 Tasty Tales. The Wild Women Association. Berkeley, Calif.: Conari Press, 1996. Great fun, this little book combines a wide range of recipes with lots of historical anecdotes.

Written by Herself. Jill Ker Conway, ed. New York: Vintage Books, 1992. This is an edited volume of women's biographical writing through history. Many moving and inspiring passages.

Videos

Videos specifically about menopause are now out of date because of the new research. Here are some on other issues we've covered.

Collage Video's Guide to Exercise Videos. This is a great resource—a catalogue that reviews and details exercise and yoga videos. It rates them by difficulty level also. 800-433 6769.

Healing and the Mind. Bill Moyers. See previous book description.

Kathy Smith's Moving Through Menopause. An exercise video for midlife women only.

Loretta Laroche Humor Your Stress. Pretty funny. Laroche has appeared on PBS programs.

Mindfulness and Meditation Stress Reduction. Jon Kabat-Zinn. Kabat-Zinn created a medication program for people with chronic pain in a major medical school. He is an engaging, comforting, good teacher.

Organizations

All of these offer free information to the public.

American Association of Clinical Endocrinologists
701 Fiasco Street, Suite 100
Jacksonville, FL 32204
904-353-7878

American Association of Sex Educators, Counselors and Therapists (AASECT)
PO Box 238
Mount Vernon, IA 52314
319-895-8407

American Cancer Society
To contact your local affiliate check the Web site—www.cancer.org—or call 1-800-ACS-2345.

American College of Obstetricians and Gynecologists (ACOG)
409 12th Street, SW
Washington, DC 20024
800-673-8444

American College of Physicians
Headquarters:
190 N Independence Mall West
Philadelphia, PA 19106-1572

Washington Office:
2011 Pennsylvania Avenue NW, Suite 800
Washington, DC 20006-1837
202-261-4500
800-338-2746

Customer Service:
800-523-1546, x2600
215-351-2600

American Heart Association
7320 Greenville Avenue
Dallas, TX 75231
214-373-6300

American Psychiatric Association
14 K Street, NW
Washington, DC 20005
202-682-6000

American Psychological Association
1200 17th Street, NW
Washington, DC 20036
800-964-2000

Association of Women's Health Obstetrics and Neonatal Nurses
2000 L Street, NW, Suite 740
Washington, DC 20036
202-261-2436

Canadian Mental Health Association
2160 Yonge Street, 3rd Floor
Toronto, Ontario M4S 2Z3
416-484-7750

Canadian Psychiatric Association
237 Argyle Avenue, Suite 200
Ottawa, Ontario K2P 1B8
613-234-2815

The Heart and Stroke Foundation of Canada
160 George Street, Suite 200
Ottawa, Ontario K1N 9M2
613-241-4361

Help for Incontinent People
PO Box 544
Union, SC 29379
800-BLADDER

National Association of Social Workers
7981 Eastern Avenue
Silver Spring, MD 20910
301-565-0333

National Association of Women's Health Professionals
816 Elmwood
Wilmette, IL 60091

National Heart, Lung, and Blood Institute
9000 Rockville Pike
Building 31, Room 4A-21
Bethesda, MD 20892
301-952-3260

National Institute of Mental Health
56000 Fishers Lane
Public Inquiries Office Room 15C-05
Rockville, MD 20857
301-443-4513

National Osteoporosis Foundation
1150 17th Street, NW, Suite 500
Washington, DC 20004
800-223-9994

National Women's Health Network
514 10th Street, NW, Suite 400
Washington, DC 20004
202-628-7814

North American Menopause Society
PO Box 94527
Cleveland, OH 44101
440-442-7550

Osteoporosis Society of Canada
33 Laird Drive
Toronto, Ontario M4G 3S9
416-696-2663

Sexuality Information and Education Council of the U.S. (SIECUS)
130 West 42nd Street, Suite 350
New York, NY 10036
212-819-9770

The Sex Information and Education Council of Canada (SIECCAN)
850 Coxwell Avenue
East York, Ontario M4C 5R1
416-466-5304

The Simon Foundation for Continence
PO Box 815
Wilmette, IL 60091
800-23-SIMON
or
PO Box 66524
Cavendish Mall P.O.
Cote St. Luc. PQ H4W 3J6
800-265-9575

The Society for Menstrual Cycle Research
President, Joan Chrysler
Department of Psychology
Connecticut College
New London, CT 06320
860-439-2336

The Society of Obstetricians and Gynaecologists of Canada (SOGC)
774 Promenade Echo Drive
Ottawa, Ontario K1S 5N8
613-730-4192

References

Chapter One. The New Truth About Menopause

Brody, J.E. "Sorting Through the Confusion Over Estrogen." *New York Times*, September 3, 2002, page F–1.

Brody, J.E. "The Search for Alternatives to Hormone Replacement Therapy." *New York Times*, September 3, 2002, page F–5.

Deutsch, H. *Psychology of Women*, Vol. 2. New York: Grune & Stratton, 1945, page 461.

Grady, D. "Hormone Use Found to Raise Dementia Risk." *New York Times*, May 28, 2003, page A–1.

Grady, D. "Hot Flashes: Exploring the Mystery of Women's Thermal Chaos." *New York Times*, September 3, 2002, page F–5.

Healy, B. "The Mysteries of Menopause." *U.S. News and World Report* 133: 39–41 (November 18, 2002).

Jabour, A. *Marriage in the Early Republic: Elizabeth and William Wirt and the Companionate Ideal*. Baltimore, Md.: Johns Hopkins Press, 2002.

Kolata, G. "Study Is Halted Over Rise Seen in Cancer Risk." *New York Times*, July 9, 2002, page A–1.

Landau, C., M.G. Cyr, and A.W. Moulton. *The Complete Book of Menopause: Every Woman's Guide to Good Health*. New York: Putnam, 1994.

Mahowald, M. "Beyond Motherhood: Ethical Issues." *Proceedings of the Third Annual Meeting of the North American Menopause Society*. Cleveland, Ohio: North American Menopause Society, 1992.

Reuben, D.R. *Everything You Always Wanted to Know About Sex, but Were Afraid to Ask, Explained by David R. Reuben*. New York: Bantam Books, 1971.

Rose, P. "Endometrial Carcinoma." *New England Journal of Medicine* 335: 640–49 (1996).

Rowan, T.C., et al. "Influence of Estrogen Plus Progestin on Breast Cancer and Mammography in Healthy Postmenopausal Women." *Journal of the American Medical Association* 289: 3243-53 (2003).

Sheehy, G. *The Silent Passage*. New York: Random House, 1991.

Sherwin, B-B. "Estrogen and Cognitive Aging in Women." *Trends in Pharmacological Science* 23(11): 527–34 (November 2002).

Shumaker, S.A., et al. "Estrogen Plus Progestin and the Incidence of Dementia and Mild Cognitive Impairment in Postmenopausal Women. The Women's Health Initiative Memory Study: A Randomized Controlled Trial." *Journal of the American Medical Association* 289: 2651–62 (2003).

Spake, A. "The Menopausal Marketplace." *U.S. News and World Report* 133: 42–50 (November 18, 2002).

Tanner, L. "Hormone-Taking Is Linked to Dementia." Associated Press, cited in yahoo health news. http://story.news.yahoo.com/news?tmpl=story&u=/ap_on_he_me/hormones_dementia. May 27, 2003.

Wilson, R. *Feminine Forever* New York: M. Evans, 1966.

Chapter Two. The Rise and Fall of Estrogen

Collaborative Group on Hormonal Factors in Breast Cancer. "Breast Cancer and Hormone Replacement Therapy: Collaborative Reanalysis of Data from 51 Epidemiological Studies of 52,705 Women with Breast Cancer and 108,411 Women Without Breast Cancer." *Lancet* 350: 1047–59 (1997).

Gambacciani, M., et al. "Effects of Low-Dose Continuous Combined Conjugated Estrogens and Medroxyprogesterone Acetate on Menopausal Symptoms, Body Weight, Bone Density, and Metabolism in Postmenopausal Women." *American Journal of Obstetrics and Gynecology* 185: 1180–85 (2001).

Gardanne, C.P.L. de. *De la ménépausie ou de l'age critique des femmes.* Paris: Chez Mequignon, Marvis Libraire, 1821.

Gass, M.L.S., and W.H. Utian and NAMS Advisory Panel. "Amended Report from the NAMS Advisory Panel on Hormone Therapy." *Menopause* 10(1): 6–12 (2003).

Grady, D, et al., for the HERS Research Group. "Cardiovascular Disease Outcomes During 6.8 Years of Hormone Therapy: Heart and Estrogen/Progestin Replacement Study Follow-up (HERS II)." *Journal of the American Medical Association* 288: 49–57 (2002).

Greenblatt, R.B. "Estrogen Therapy for Post-Menopausal Females." *New England Journal of Medicine* 272: 305–308 (1965).

Grodstein, F., et al. "A Prospective, Observational Study of Postmenopausal Hormone Therapy and Primary Prevention of Cardiovascular Disease." *Annals of Internal Medicine* 133: 933–41 (2000).

Grodstein, F., et al. "Post-Menopausal Hormone Therapy and Mortality." *New England Journal of Medicine* 336: 1769–75 (1997).

Grodstein, F., et al. "Post-Menopausal Estrogen and Progestin Use and the Risk of Cardiovascular Disease." *New England Journal of Medicine* 335: 453–61 (1996).

Herrington, D.M., et al., for the HERS Study Group. "Statin Therapy, Cardiovascular Events and Total Mortality in the Heart and Estrogen/Progestin Replacement Study (HERS)." *Circulation* 105: 2962–67 (2002).

Hsia, J., et al. "Peripheral Arterial Disease in Randomized Trial of Estrogen with Progestin in Women with Coronary Heart Disease: The Heart and Estrogen/Progestin Replacement Study." *Circulation* 102: 2228–32 (2000).

Hulley, S., et al., for the Heart and Estrogen/Progestin Replacement Study (HERS) Research Group. "Randomized Trial of Estrogen Plus Progestin for Secondary Prevention of Coronary Heart Disease in Postmenopausal Women." *Journal of the American Medical Association* 280: 605–13 (1998).

Keating, N.L., et al. "Use of Hormone Replacement Therapy by Postmenopausal Women in the United States." *Annals of Internal Medicine* 130: 545–53 (1999).

Lacey, J.V., et al. "Menopausal Hormone Replacement Therapy and Risk of Ovarian Cancer." *Journal of the American Medical Association* 288: 334–41 (2002).

LeBlanc, E.S., et al. "Hormone Replacement Therapy and Cognition: Systematic Review and Meta-Analysis." *Journal of the American Medical Association* 285: 1489–99 (2001).

Menopause in 1903. www.geocities.com/menobeyond/1903/html. Viewed February 16, 2003.

National Association of Nurse Practitioners in Women's Health. "Hormone Replacement Therapy: Guidance from the National Association of Nurse Practitioners in Women's Health." Topics in Advanced Practice Nursing eJournal 2(3): Medscape (2002).

Pierce, R.V. *The People's Common Sense Medical Adviser in Plain English.* Buffalo, N.Y.: World's Dispensary Printing Office and Bindery, 1895.

Rapp, S.R., et al. "Effect of Estrogen Plus Progestin on Global Cognitive Function in Postmenopausal Women. The Women's Health Initiative Memory Study: A Randomized Controlled Trial." *Journal of the American Medical Association* 289: 2663–72 (2003).

Reuben, D.R. *Everything You Always Wanted to Know About Sex, but Were Afraid to Ask, Explained by David R. Reuben.* New York: Bantam Books, 1971.

Rowan, T.C., et al. "Influence of Estrogen Plus Progestin on Breast Cancer and Mammography in Healthy Postmenopausal Women." *Journal of the American Medical Association* 289: 3243-53 (2003).

Schairer, C., et al. "Menopausal Estrogen and Estrogen-Progestin Replacement Therapy and Breast Cancer Risk." *Journal of the American Medical Association* 283: 485–91 (2000).

Shumaker, S.A., et al. "Estrogen Plus Progestin and the Incidence of Dementia and Mild Cognitive Impairment in Postmenopausal Women. The Women's Health Initiative Memory Study: A Randomized Controlled Trial." *Journal of the American Medical Association* 289: 2651–62 (2003).

Simon, J.A., et al. "Postmenopausal Hormone Therapy and Risk of Stroke: The Heart and Estrogen-Progestin Replacement Study (HERS)." *Circulation* 103: 638–42 (2001).

Sith, D.C., et al. "Association of Exogenous Estrogen and Endometrial Carcinoma." *New England Journal of Medicine* 293: 1164–67 (1975).

Spake, A. "The Menopausal Marketplace." *U.S. News and World Report* 133: 42–50 (November 18, 2002).

Speroff, L. "The Impact of the Women's Health Initiative on Clinical Practice." *Journal of the Society for Gynecological Investigation* 9(5): 251–53 (2002).

Walsh, A. *ERT: The Pills to Keep Women Young.* Ojai, Calif.: Edwin Publishing Company, 1965.

Wassertheil-Smoller, S., et al. "Effect of Estrogen Plus Progestin on Stroke in Postmenopausal Women. The Women's Health Initiative: A Randomized Trial." *Journal of the American Medical Association* 289: 2673–84 (2003).

Wilson, R. *Feminine Forever.* New York: M. Evans and Co., 1966.

Writing Group for the Women's Health Initiative Investigators. "Risks and Benefits of Estrogen Plus Progestin in Healthy Postmenopausal Women: Principal Results from the Women's Health Initiative Randomized Controlled Trial." *Journal of the American Medical Association* 288: 321–33 (2002).

Yaffe, K., et al. "Estrogen Therapy in Postmenopausal Women: Effects on Cognitive Function and Dementia." *Journal of the American Medical Association* 279: 688–95 (1998).

Yaffe, K., et al. "Hormone Therapy and the Brain: Déjà Vu All Over Again?" *Journal of the American Medical Association* 289: 2727–19 (2003).

Ziel, H.K., and W.D. Finkle. "Increased Risk of Endometrial Carcinoma Among Users of Conjugated Estrogens." *New England Journal of Medicine* 293: 1167–70 (1975).

Chapter Three. Treating the Symptoms of Menopause

"Adding Soy Protein to Diet." FDA Consumer, www.cfsan.fda.gov/~dms/fdsoypr.html.

Avis, N-E., et al. "Longitudinal Study of Hormone Levels and Depression Among Women Transitioning Through Menopause." *Climacteric* 4(3): 243–49 (September 2001).

Avlimil Web site, www.avlimil.com.

Barton, D.L., et al. "Prospective Evaluation of Vitamin E for Hot Flashes in Breast Cancer Survivors." *Journal of Clinical Oncology* 16: 495–500 (1998).

Boosting Bone Strength: A Guide to Preventing and Treating Osteoporosis. Harvard Health Publications, Boston, 2000.

FDA Consumer. "Soy: Health Claims for Soy Protein, Questions About Other Components." www.cfsan.fda.gov/~dms/fdsoypr.html.

Fitzpatrick, L.A., and R.J. Santen. "Hot Flashes: The Old and the New, What Is Really True?" *Mayo Clinic Proceedings* 77: 1155–58 (2002).

Gass, M., and M. Taylor. "Alternatives for Women Through Menopause." *American Journal of Obstetrics and Gynecology* 185: S47–S56 (2001).

Grady, D., et al. "Postmenopausal Hormone Therapy Increases Risk for Venous Thromboembolic Disease." *Annals of Internal Medicine* 132: 689–96 (2000).

Guttuso, T.J. "Gabapentin's Effects on Hot Flashes and Hypothermia." *Neurology* 54: 2161–63 (2000).

Hlatky, M.A., et al. for the Heart and Estrogen/Progestin Replacement Study (HERS) Research Group. "Quality-of-life and Depressive Symptoms in Post-menopausal Women After Receiving Hormone Therapy: Results from the Heart and Estrogen/Progestin Replacement Study (HERS) Trial." *Journal of the American Medical Association* 287: 591–97 (2002).

Jacobson, J.S., et al. "Randomized Trial of Black Cohosh for the Treatment of Hot Flashes Among Women with a History of Breast Cancer." *Journal of Clinical Oncology* 19: 2739–45 (2001).

Kronenberg, F., and A. Fugh-Berman. "Complementary and Alternative Medicine for Menopausal Symptoms: A Review of Randomized, Controlled Trials." *Annals of Internal Medicine* 137: 805–13 (2002).

Landau, C., and F. B. Milan. "Assessment and Treatment of Depression During the Menopause: A Preliminary Report." *Menopause* 3(4): 201–207 (1996).

Leonetti, H.B., S. Longo, and J.N. Anasti. "Transdermal Progesterone Cream for Vasomotor Symptoms and Postmenopausal Bone Loss." *Obstetrics and Gynecology* 94(2): 225–28 (1999).

Loprinzi, C.L., et al. "Megestrol Acetate for the Prevention of Hot Flashes." *New England Journal of Medicine* 331: 347–52 (1994).

Loprinzi, C.L., et al. "Phase III Evaluation of Fluoxetine for Treatment of Hot Flashes." *Journal of Clinical Oncology* 20: 1578–83 (2002).

Loprinzi, C.L., et al. "Pilot Evaluation of Gabapentin for Treating Hot Flashes." *Mayo Clinic Proceedings* 77: 1159–63 (2002)

Loprinzi, C.L., et al. "Venlafaxine in Management of Hot Flashes in Survivors of Breast Cancer: A Randomized Controlled Trial." *Lancet* 356: 2059–63 (2000).

Managing Osteoporosis, Part 3: Prevention and Treatment of Postmenopausal Osteoporosis. American Medical Association, 2000.

McKinlay, J, S McKinlay, and D. Brambilla. "The Relative Contributions of Endocrine Changes and Social Circumstances to Depression in Mid-Aged Women." *Journal of Health and Social Behavior* 28: 345–63 (December 1987).

Michael, A., and J.J. Herrod. "Citalopram-Induced Decreased Libido." *British Journal of Psychiatry* 171: 90 (July 1997).

Montejo, A.L., et al. "Incidence of Sexual Dysfunction Associated with Antidepressant Agents: A Prospective Multicenter Study of 1022 Outpatients." Spanish Working Group for the Study of Psychotropic-Related Sexual Dysfunction. *Journal of Clinical Psychiatry* 62 (Suppl. 3): 10–21 (2001).

North American Menopause Society. *Menopause Core Curriculum Study Guide*, 2nd ed. Cleveland, Ohio: North American Menopause Society, 2002

Osteoporosis: Guide to Prevention, Diagnosis and Treatment. Boston: Brigham and Women's Hospital, 2002.

Pandya, K.J., et al. "Oral Clonidine in Postmenopausal Patients with Breast Cancer Experiencing Tamoxifen-Induced Hot Flashes." *Annals of Internal Medicine* 132: 788–93 (2000).

Quella, S.K., et al. "Evaluation of Soy Phytoestrogens for the Treatment of Hot Flashes in Breast Cancer Survivors: A North Central Cancer Treatment Group Trial." *Journal of Clinical Oncology* 18: 1068–74 (2000).

Rowan, T.C., et al. "Influence of Estrogen Plus Progestin on Breast Cancer and Mammography in Healthy Postmenopausal Women." *Journal of the American Medical Association* 289: 3243-53 (2003).

Shen, W.W. "Sildenafil in the Treatment of Female Sexual Dysfunction Induced by Selective Serotonin Reuptake Inhibitors." *Journal of Reproductive Medicine* 44(6): 535–42 (1999).

Sherwin, B-B. "Estrogen and Cognitive Aging in Women." *Trends in Pharmacological Science* 23(11): 527–34 (November 2002).

Stearns, V., et al. "A Pilot Trial Assessing the Efficacy of Paroxetine Hydrochloride (Paxil) in Controlling Hot Flashes in Breast Cancer Survivors." *Annals of Oncology* 11: 17–22 (2000).

Willett, W.C., and M.J. Stampfer. "What Vitamins Should I Be Taking, Doctor?" *New England Journal of Medicine* 345 (25): 1819–24 (2001).

Chapter Four. Strong Bones and Healthy Hearts

Barrett-Connor, E., et al. "Raloxifene and Cardiovascular Events in Osteoporotic Postmenopausal Women." *Journal of the American Medical Association* 287: 847–57 (2002).

Cummings, S.R., et al. "The Effect of Raloxifene on Risk of Breast Cancer in Postmenopausal Women: Results from the MORE Randomized Trial. Multiple Outcomes of Raloxifene Evaluation." *Journal of the American Medical Association* 281: 2189–98 (1999).

Cyr, M.G., and K.A. McGarry. "Alcohol Use Disorders in Women: Screening Methods and Approaches to Treatment." *Postgraduate Medicine* 112(6): 31–47 (2002).

Davidson, K., et al. "Constructive Anger Verbal Behavior Predicts Blood Pressure in a Population-Based Sample." *Health Psychology* 19: 55–64 (2002).

Denollet, J. "Personality and Coronary Heart Disease: the Type-D Scale-16 (DS16)." *Annals of Behavioral Medicine* 20(3): 209–15 (Summer 1998).

Denollet, J. "Type D Personality. A Potential Risk Factor Refined." *Journal of Psychosomatic Research* 49(4): 255–66 (2000).

Denollet, J., et al. "Personality as Independent Predictor of Long-Term Mortality in Patients with Coronary Heart Disease." *Lancet* 347(8999): 417–21 (February 1996).

Grady, D., et al. "Cardiovascular Disease Outcomes During 6.8 Years of Hormone Therapy: Heart and Estrogen/Progestin Replacement Study Follow-Up (HERS II)." *Journal of the American Medical Association* 288: 49 (2002).

Hulley, S., et al. "Randomized Trial of Estrogen Plus Progestin for Secondary Prevention of Coronary Heart Disease in Postmenopausal Women." *Journal of the American Medical Association* 280: 605–13 (1998).

North American Menopause Society. *Menopause Core Curriculum Study Guide,* 2nd ed. Cleveland, Ohio: North American Menopause Society, 2002.

Peck, P. "C-Reactive Protein Testing Endorsed for Limited Use." *Internal Medicine News* 36(4): 1–2 (2003).

Siris, E.S., et al. "Identification and Fracture Outcomes of Undiagnosed Low Bone Mineral Density in Postmenopausal Women." *Journal of the American Medical Association* 285: 2815–55 (2001).

Smith, D. "Angry Thoughts, At-Risk Hearts." *Monitor on Psychology,* March 2003, pages 46–48.

Smith, T.W., and L.C. Gallo. "Hostility and Cardiovascular Reactivity During Marital Interaction." *Psychosomatic Medicine* 6: 436–45 (1999).

Suarez, E.C., et al. "Cardiovascular and Emotional Responses in Women: The Role of Hostility and Harassment." *Health Psychology* 12: 459–68 (1993).

Sullivan, J.M., and L.P. Fowlkes. "The Clinical Aspects of Estrogen and the Cardiovascular System." *Obstetrics and Gynecology* 87: 36S–43S (1996).

Writing Group for the PEPI Trial. "The Effects of Estrogen or Estrogen/Progestin Regimens on Heart Disease Risk Factors in Postmenopausal Women." *Journal of the American Medical Association* 273: 199–208 (1995).

"Your Heart Risk: Inflammation Counts." *Harvard Women's Health Watch,* February 2003, pages 1–2.

Chapter Five. Not Your Average Menopause

Bultz, B.D., et al. "A Randomized Controlled Trial of a Brief Psychoeducational Support Group for Partners of Early Stage Breast Cancer Patients." *Psychooncology* 9: 303–13 (2002).

Burstein, H.J., and E.P. Winer. "Primary Care for Survivors of Breast Cancer." *New England Journal of Medicine* 343: 1086–94 (2000).

Carlson, K.C., D.H. Nichols, and I. Schiff. "Indications for Hysterectomy." *New England Journal of Medicine* 328: 856–60 (1993).

Col, N.F., et al. "Hormone Replacement Therapy After Breast Cancer: A Systematic Review and Quantitative Assessment of Risk." *Journal of Clinical Oncology* 19: 2357–63 (2001).

Coughlin, S.S., et al. "A Meta-Analysis of Estrogen Replacement Therapy and Risk of Epithelial Ovarian Cancer." *Journal of Clinical Epidemiology* 53: 367–75 (2000).

Epstein, R.H. "Sifting Through the Online Medical Jumble." *New York Times*, Health & Fitness Section, January 28, 2003.

Garge, P.P., et al. "Hormone Replacement Therapy and the Risk for Epithelial Ovarian Carcinoma: A Meta-Analysis." *Obstetrics and Gynecology* 92: 472–79 (1998).

Kesharvarz, H., et al. "Hysterectomy Surveillance—United States 1994–1999." Center for Disease Control, *Morbidity and Mortality Weekly Report* 51(SS05): 1–8 (July 12, 2002).

McKinlay, J., S. McKinlay, and D. Brambilla. "The Relative Contributions of Endocrine Changes and Social Circumstances to Depression in Mid-Aged Women." *Journal of Health and Social Behavior* 28: 345–63 (December 1987).

Osborne, C.K. "Tamoxifen in the Treatment of Breast Cancer." *New England Journal of Medicine* 339: 1609–18 (1998).

Rannestad, T., et al. "The General Health in Women Suffering from Gynecological Disorders Is Improved by Means of Hysterectomy." *Scandinavian Journal of Caring Sciences* 15: 264–70 (2001).

Reed, G., and J. Spira. "Group Psychotherapy for Women with Breast Cancer." American Psychological Association, 2003.

Sands, R., et al. "Current Opinion: Hormone Replacement Therapy After a Diagnosis of Breast Cancer." *Menopause: The Journal of the North American Menopause Society* 2: 73–80 (1995).

Chapter Six. Communicating with Your Doctor About Your Health

Lazare, A. "Shame and Humiliation in the Medical Encounter." *Archives of Internal Medicine* 147: 1653–58 (1987).

Marvel, M.K., et al. "Soliciting the Patient's Agenda: Have We Improved?" *Journal of the American Medical Association* 281: 283–87 (1999).

Roter, D.L., and J.A. Hall. *Doctors Talking with Patients/Patients Talking with Doctors: Improving Communication in Medical Visits.* Westport, Conn.: Auburn House, 1993.

Shorter, E. *Doctors and Their Patients: A Social History.* Somerset, N.J.: Transaction Publications, 1991.

Chapter Seven. Making a Plan

Cummings, S.R., et al. "The Effect of Raloxifene on Risk of Breast Cancer in Postmenopausal Women: Results from the MORE Randomized Trial. Multiple Outcomes of Raloxifene Evaluation." *Journal of the American Medical Association* 281: 2189–98 (1999).

"Facts About Postmenopausal Hormone Therapy." National Heart, Lung and Blood Institute, http://www.nhlbi.nih.gov/health/women/pht_facts.htm.

Hlatky, M.A., et al. for the Heart and Estrogen/Progestin Replacement Study (HERS) Research Group. "Quality-of-life and Depressive Symptoms in Postmenopausal Women After Receiving Hormone Therapy: Results from the Heart and Estrogen/Progestin Replacement Study (HERS) Trial." *Journal of the American Medical Association* 287: 591–97 (2002).

Landau, C., F.B. Milan, and I. Shuey. "Depressive Disorders." In K.J. Carlson and S.A. Eisenstat, eds., *Primary Care of Women,* 2nd ed. St. Louis: Mosby Press, 2002.

Chapter Eight. Is the Plan Working?

"Combination HRT Not for Long-Term Use." Special Report on Women's Health in *Primary Care* 5: 491–92 (August 2002).

Cummings, S.R., et al. "The Effect of Raloxifene on Risk of Breast Cancer in Postmenopausal Women: Results from the MORE Randomized Trial. Multiple Outcomes of Raloxifene Evaluation." *Journal of the American Medical Association* 281: 2189–98 (1999).

Loprinzi, C.L., et al. "Phase III Evaluation of Fluovetine for Treatment of Hot Flashes." *Journal of Clinical Oncology* 20: 1578–83 (2002).

Loprinzi, C.L., et al. "Pilot Evaluation of Gabapentin for Treating Hot Flashes." *Mayo Clinic Proceedings* 77: 1159–63 (2002).

Loprinzi, C.L., et al. "Venlafaxine in Management of Hot Flashes in Survivors of Breast Cancer: A Randomized Controlled Trial." *Lancet* 356: 2059–63 (2000).

Pradhan, A.D., et al. "Inflammatory Biomarkers, Hormone Replacement Therapy, and Incident Coronary Heart Disease: Prospective Analysis from the Women's Health Initiative Observational Study." *Journal of the American Medical Association* 288(8): 980–87 (2002).

Rowan, T.C., et al. "Influence of Estrogen Plus Progestin on Breast Cancer and Mammography in Healthy Postmenopausal Women." *Journal of the American Medical Association* 289: 3243-53 (2003).

Writing Group for the Women's Health Initiative Investigators. "Risks and Benefits of Estrogen Plus Progestin in Healthy Postmenopausal Women: Principal Results from the Women's Health Initiative Randomized Controlled Trial." *Journal of the American Medical Association* 288: 321–33 (2002).

Chapter Nine: Creative Thoughts and Strong Bonds

American Cancer Society. *Cancer Facts and Figures.* Atlanta, Georgia, 2002.

Bassuk, S.S., T.A. Glass, and L.F. Berkman. "Social Disengagement and Incident Cognitive Decline in Community Dwelling Elderly Persons." *Annals of Internal Medicine* 131:165–73 (1999).

Brown, G.W., and T. Harris. *Social Origins of Depression.* New York: Free Press, 1978.

Fingerman, K.L., and P.C. Griffiths. "Season's Greetings: Adults' Social Contacts at the Holiday Season." *Psychology of Aging* 14: 192–205 (1999).

"Gender and Stress." *Harvard Women's Health Watch.* October 1999, page 1.

Gottman, J. *Seven Principles for Making Marriage Work.* New York: Crown, 1999.

Haynes, R.B., H. Feinleib, and W.B. Kannel. "The Relationship of Psychosocial Factors to Coronary Heart Disease in the Framingham Study: Eight-Year Incidence of Coronary Heart Disease." *American Journal of Epidemiology* 11: 37–58 (1980).

Jack, D.C. *The Silencing of the Self.* New York: HarperCollins, 1993.

Kayser, K., M. Sormanti, and E. Strainchamps. "Women Coping with Cancer: The Influence of Relationship Factors on Psychosocial Adjustment." *Psychology of Women Quarterly* 1999: 725–39 (1999).

Landau, C., M.G. Cyr, and A.W. Moulton. *The Complete Book of Menopause: Every Woman's Guide to Good Health.* New York: Putnam, 1994.

Lundberg, U. "Influence of Paid and Unpaid Employment on Psycho-physiological Stress." *Journal of Occupational Health* 1: 117–40 (1996).

Nolen-Hoeksema, S. *Sex Differences in Depression.* Palo Alto, Calif.: Stanford University Press, 1990.

Nolen-Hoeksema, S. "Sex Differences in Unipolar Depression: Evidence and Theory." *Psychological Bulletin* 101: 259–82 (1987).

Tyler, A. *Back When We Were Grownups.* New York: Ballantine Books, 2002.

Acknowledgments

We have been fortunate to work with many gifted and collaborative colleagues. Our friend and coauthor of *The Complete Book of Menopause*, Anne W. Moulton, M.D., is always generous with her ideas and her time.

Drs. Karen Carlson, Nananda Col, Barbara McCrady, Kelly McGarry, Janice Prochaska, and Diana Taylor have made helpful comments and suggestions.

We would also like to thank Eileen Richter for her assistance with research and Heather Florence for her advice.

We thank our supportive friends and extended families, the Landau, Ames, Cyr, and Towne families. Also Pat Baum, Dorothy Bianco, Betty Fielder, Rosemarie Helmbrecht, Caroline Fields, Williams Fields, Belinda Johnson, Carol Levine, David Levine, Iris Shuey, and Michael Stein.

We are grateful to our agent, Joelle Delbourgo, and our editor, Hope Dellon, as well as Kris Kamikawa at St. Martin's Press.

This book would not have been possible without the administrative skills, dedication, and wit of Michael J. Chamberlain.

Many thanks to all.

Index

daidzein, 46
daily requirements, 66
dairy products, 65–66
dementia, 2
  prevention, 31
  risk of, 31, 34
depression
  case study, 120–21
  medical causes of, 82, 87–89
  menopause and, 58, 88
  midlife, 8, 13–14, 138–39
  treatment of, 45, 58–60, 134
  in younger women, 14
Deutsch, Helene, 8
diabetes mellitus, 77
diagnostic procedures, 98
diary
  of menopausal symptoms, 41, 101, 112
  using to assess a plan, 125
DiClemente, Carlo, 72
diet, and health, 78, 130
dieting, diets, 78–80
  extreme, 65
  fad, 65
  high-protein (Atkins), 78
  low-fat (Ornish), 78
Discovery Channel, 148
diuretics, 76
doctor
  anger at, 117, 131
  asking one for a medical recommendation, 100–101
  checklist for appointment, 106
  choosing a primary care physician, 99
  communication, 17, 96–98, 101, 151
  looking for a new one, 105
  male vs. female, 99
Doisy, Edward, 22
dong quai, 43
"doorknob" comments, 104–5
double-blind study, 29
douching, 50
drinking, moderate, 77–78
drugs. *See* medications
dry milk, powdered, 66
dual energy X-ray absorptiometry (DEXA), 69
dyspareunia, 50

education, resuming in midlife, 141
educational institutions, social support from, 146
Effexor, 45, 121
eggs, human female, 7
ejaculation, premature, 24
Elavil, 60
e-mail communication with doctor, 98
Emmenin, 22
endometrial biopsies, 127
endometrial hyperplasia, 6, 26, 85, 127
endometriosis, 86
  hysterectomy as treatment for, 85
EPT. *See* estrogen plus progestin therapy
erectile dysfunction, 5, 55
Erickson, Erik, 140
estradiol, 7, 50
estradiol/progestin patch, 127
Estratest, 56
Estring, 50
estrogen, 6, 7
  benefits, 28
  decreased production, 7
  forms, 40
  levels, 39
  sales, 4
  studies, 27, 29–33
  systemic use, 124
  topical, vaginal use, 49, 124
  unopposed, 127
estrogen plus progestin therapy (EPT; HT; HRT), 6
  benefits, 26, 27–30, 59
  dangers, 1–2, 34, 123
  invention of, 26
  number of prescriptions, 29
  pros and cons, 31, 122–24
  reducing gradually, 123
  short-term, 116, 128
  studies, 1, 33
estrogen replacement therapy. *See* estrogen therapy
estrogen ring, 93
estrogen therapy (ET; ERT), 6, 39–41
  benefits, 59, 61
  dangers, 22, 26, 29
  after hysterectomy, 29, 40, 87
  vaginal use, 53
estrone, 7
  discovery, 22

About the Authors

Carol Landau, Ph.D., is clinical professor of psychiatry and human behavior at Brown Medical School. Dr. Landau maintains an independent practice of consultation and psychotherapy. She is also chair of the behavioral sciences committee in the division of general internal medicine at Rhode Island Hospital and Brown Medical School. She has written numerous articles and chapters on women's psychological issues. Dr. Landau is on the medical advisory board of the Wellness Councils of America and has served on the education committee of the North American Menopause Society.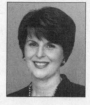

Michele G. Cyr, M.D., F.A.C.P., currently serves as the director of the division of general internal medicine, associate dean of graduate medical education, and associate professor of medicine at Brown Medical School. Dr. Cyr is also the program director for the general internal medicine residency at Rhode Island Hospital. Dr. Cyr has written numerous articles, reviews, and chapters on women's health topics and is a regular presenter at the meetings of the American College of Physicians. She is the recipient of more than fifteen postgraduate honors and awards, including Rhode Island's Outstanding Woman in Science Award in 2001. In addition, she is coprincipal investigator for the Women's Health Initiative Vanguard Center at Memorial Hospital of Rhode Island.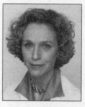

Dr. Landau and Dr. Cyr, together with Anne W. Moulton, M.D., wrote *The Complete Book of Menopause: Every Woman's Guide to Good Health*, an award-winning text selected by *Prevention* magazine and *Consumer Reports* for their book clubs. They also served for seven years as monthly contributors to "The Doctors Are In" column for *McCall's* magazine. With Dr. Moulton, they cofounded the Women's Health Associates, a comprehensive group practice affiliated with Rhode Island Hospital and Brown Medical School. They have served on the faculty of the Harvard Medical School continuing education course "The Primary Care of Women," and they deliver national seminars and lectures on menopause and women's health.